# THE WASHINGTON MANUAL™ OF ECHOCARDIOGRAPHY

*Editor*

**Ravi Rasalingam,** MD, FACC
Assistant Professor of Medicine
Division of Cardiology
Washington University School of Medicine
St. Louis, Missouri

*Associate Editors*

**Majesh Makan,** MD, FACC, FASE
Associate Professor of Medicine
Associate Director of Echocardiography
Washington University School of Medicine
St. Louis, Missouri

**Julio E. Pérez,** MD, FACC, FAHA, FASE, FACP
Professor of Medicine
Director of Echocardiography
Washington University School of Medicine
St. Louis, Missouri

 Wolters Kluwer | Lippincott Williams & Wilkins
Health

Philadelphia • Baltimore • New York • London
Buenos Aires • Hong Kong • Sydney • Tokyo

*Acquisitions Editor:* Julie Goolsby
*Product Manager:* Leanne Vandetty
*Production Manager:* Bridgett Dougherty
*Senior Manufacturing Manager:* Benjamin Rivera
*Marketing Manager:* Kimberly Schonberger
*Design Coordinator:* Stephen Druding
*Production Service:* Aptara, Inc.

**© 2013 by Department of Medicine, Washington University School of Medicine**

Printed in China

**Library of Congress Cataloging-in-Publication Data**

The Washington manual of echocardiography / editor, Ravi Rasalingam ; associate editors, Majesh Makan, Julio E. Pérez.
    p. ; cm.
  Echocardiography
  Includes bibliographical references and index.
    ISBN 978-1-4511-1340-2 (pbk. : alk. paper) — ISBN 1-4511-1340-4 (pbk. : alk. paper)
  I. Rasalingam, Ravi. II. Makan, Majesh. III. Pérez, Julio E. IV. Washington University (Saint Louis, Mo.). School of Medicine. V. Title: Echocardiography.
  [DNLM: 1. Echocardiography—methods. 2. Heart Diseases—ultrasonography. WG 141.5.E2]

  616.1′207543–dc23

                                                                                    2012017203

Care has been taken to confirm the accuracy of the information presented and to describe generally accepted practices. However, the authors, editors, and publisher are not responsible for errors or omissions or for any consequences from application of the information in this book and make no warranty, expressed or implied, with respect to the currency, completeness, or accuracy of the contents of the publication. Application of the information in a particular situation remains the professional responsibility of the practitioner.

The authors, editors, and publisher have exerted every effort to ensure that drug selection and dosage set forth in this text are in accordance with current recommendations and practice at the time of publication. However, in view of ongoing research, changes in government regulations, and the constant flow of information relating to drug therapy and drug reactions, the reader is urged to check the package insert for each drug for any change in indications and dosage and for added warnings and precautions. This is particularly important when the recommended agent is a new or infrequently employed drug.

Some drugs and medical devices presented in the publication have Food and Drug Administration (FDA) clearance for limited use in restricted research settings. It is the responsibility of the health care provider to ascertain the FDA status of each drug or device planned for use in their clinical practice.

To purchase additional copies of this book, call our customer service department at (800) 638-3030 or fax orders to (301) 223-2320. International customers should call (301) 223-2300.

Visit Lippincott Williams & Wilkins on the Internet: at LWW.com. Lippincott Williams & Wilkins customer service representatives are available from 8:30 am to 6 pm, EST.

10 9 8 7 6 5 4 3 2 1

CCS0712

# Dedication

To the Washington University Cardiology Fellowship Program and Barnes Jewish Hospital Cardiac Diagnostic Laboratory.

# Contributors

Suzanne V. Arnold, MD, MHA
Advanced Research Fellow
Cardiovascular Division
Washington University School of
    Medicine
St. Louis, Missouri

Sudeshna Banerjee, MD
Cardiologist
Oregon Heart & Vascular Institute
Sacred Heart Medical Center
Springfield, Oregon

Daniel H. Cooper, MD
Assistant Professor of Medicine
Cardiovascular Division
Washington University School of
    Medicine
St. Louis, Missouri

Christopher L. Holley, MD, PhD
Instructor in Medicine
Cardiovascular Division
Washington University School of
    Medicine
St. Louis, Missouri

Pei-Hsiu Huang, MD
Interventional Fellow
Cardiovascular Division
Brigham and Women's Hospital and
    Harvard Medical School
Boston, Massachusetts

Stephanie N. Johnson, RDCS
St. Louis, Missouri

Thomas K. Kurian, MD
Electrophysiology Fellow
Cardiovascular Division
Washington University School of
    Medicine
St. Louis, Missouri

Brian R. Lindman, MD
Assistant Professor of Medicine
Cardiovascular Division
Washington University School of
    Medicine
St. Louis, Missouri

Jose A. Madrazo, MD
Assistant Professor of Medicine
Cardiovascular Division
Washington University School of
    Medicine
St. Louis, Missouri

Majesh Makan, MD, FACC, FASE
Associate Professor of Medicine
Associate Director of Echocardiography
Washington University School of
    Medicine
St. Louis, Missouri

Anupama Rao, MD
Medical Officer
Division of Cardiovascular Sciences
National Heart, Lung and Blood
    Institute
Bethesda, Maryland

Ravi Rasalingam, MD, FACC
Assistant Professor of Medicine
Division of Cardiology
Washington University School of
    Medicine
St. Louis, Missouri

Mohammed K. Saghir, MD
Fellow
Cardiovascular Division
Washington University School of
   Medicine
St. Louis, Missouri

Michael Yeung, MD
Interventional Fellow
Cardiovascular Division
Washington University School of
   Medicine
St. Louis, Missouri

# Preface

*Beep! Beep! Beep!* The on-call pager signals another patient in need of cardiology consultation in the middle of the night. An echocardiogram is not an infrequent request as part of that consultation at our hospital and many others across the country. Yet, as a cardiology fellow faced with a wide array of new procedures and knowledge, the ability to adequately perform and interpret an echocardiogram remains a daunting task. There are a number of excellent, comprehensive textbooks regarding echocardiography. However, our fellows have frequently complained that there is no "handbook" that they have found useful to carry as an introduction to this field or as a reminder of the critical elements and findings of an echocardiographic examination. The primary goal of this book, therefore, has been to bridge this gap that a novice to this field experiences but also to provide succinct and useful tips that highlight the amazing depth and diagnostic utility of this modality.

Despite a challenging economic environment, the role and use of echocardiography continues to grow in the care of cardiac patients. This is related to this technique's wide availability, ease of application, lack of harmful radiation and comprehensive anatomic and hemodynamic information that is provided on a real-time basis. The technology has continued to evolve to not only increase the quality and accuracy of this information but also extend its use to practitioners outside of cardiology. The use of handheld ultrasound devices, for example, is now part of reality, and emergency departments and intensive care physicians in particular have used this technology to rapidly evaluate patients with cardiac complaints. This book will be a valuable resource for all those physicians interested in this field.

Finally, this book was conceived and written by our cardiology fellows, who have worked and trained in a busy academic hospital. In their exposure to interesting and challenging cases, they provide a unique perspective, from a trainee's point of view, as to what constitutes critical pieces of knowledge to be gained in this field. We hope that this book imparts not only this fundamental understanding of echocardiography but also an enthusiasm for further knowledge in this area.

*Ravi Rasalingam*
*Majesh Makan*
*Julio E. Pérez*

# Acknowledgments

We would like to thank the talented Washington University Cardiology fellows who participated in the development of this book. In particular, Drs. Anupama Rao and Michael Yeung for bringing the necessity of this type of textbook to our attention and their efforts in initiating this project. Our assistant, Mrs. Debbie Ermold-Taylor, was instrumental in the final stages of manuscript preparation. The echocardiographic images were performed at the Barnes-Jewish Hospital Cardiac Diagnostic Laboratory by our gifted and dedicated cardiac sonographers.

# Acknowledgments

# Contents

# Abbreviations

Acute coronary syndrome (ACS)

Anterolateral papillary muscle (ALP)

Aortic regurgitation (AR)

Aortic stenosis (AS)

Aortic valve (AoV)

Aortic valve area (AVA)

Apical five-chamber (A5C)

Apical four-chamber (A4C)

Apical long axis (APLAX)

Apical two-chamber (A2C)

Arrhythmogenic right ventricular dysplasia (ARVD)

Asymmetric septal hypertrophy (ASH)

Atrial septal defect (ASD)

Atrio-ventricular (AV)

AV canal defects (AVCD)

Bicuspid aortic valves (BAVs)

Body surface area (BSA)

Cardiac index (CI)

Cardiac output (CO)

Continuous wave Doppler (CW)

Dilated cardiomyopathy (DCM)

Effective orifice area (EOA)

Effective regurgitant orifice area (EROA)

Ejection fraction (EF)

High pulse repetition frequency (HPRF)

Hypertrophic cardiomyopathy (HCM)

Infective endocarditis (IE)

Inferior vena cava (IVC)

Intravenous (IV)

Ischemic mitral regurgitation (IMR)

Isovolumic contraction time (IVCT)

Isovolumic relaxation time (IVRT)

Left atrial appendage (LAA)

Left atrium (LA)

Left ventricle (LV)

Left ventricular (LV)

Left ventricular outflow tract (LVOT)

Mechanical index (MI)

Mitral regurgitation (MR)

Mitral stenosis (MS)

Mitral valve (MV)

Mitral valve area (MVA)

Myocardial infarction (MI)

Myocardial performance index (MPI)

Negative predictive value (NPV)

Parasternal long axis (PLAX)

Parasternal short axis (PSAX)

Patent ductus arteriosis (PDA)

Patent foramen ovale (PFO)

Patient prosthesis mismatch (PPM)

Persistent left superior vena cava (PLSVC)

Posterior-medial papillary muscle (PMP)

Pressure half time (PHT)

Proximal isovelocity surface area (PISA)

Pulmonary artery (PA)

Pulmonary artery systolic pressure (PASP)

Pulmonary capillary wedge pressure (PCWP)

Pulmonary embolism (PE)

Pulmonic stenosis (PS)

Pulmonic valve area (PVA)

Pulsed wave Doppler (PW)

Pulse repetition frequency (PRF)

Restrictive cardiomyopathy (RCM)

Right atrium (RA)

Right ventricle (RV)

Right ventricular outflow tract (RVOT)

RV inflow tract (RVIT)

RV systolic pressure (RVSP)

Sinus of Valsalva aneurysms (SVA)

Stroke volume (SV)

Superior vena cava (SVC)

Suprasternal notch (SSN)

Systolic anterior motion (SAM)

Systolic blood pressure (SBP)

Tissue Doppler imaging (TDI)
Transesophageal echocardiography (TEE)
Transthoracic echocardiography (TTE)
Tricuspid annular plane systolic excursion (TAPSE)
Tricuspid regurgitation (TR)
Tricuspid valve (TV)
Velocity time integral (VTI)
Ventricular septal defect (VSD)
Ventricular septal rupture (VSR)
Wall motion score index (WMSI)

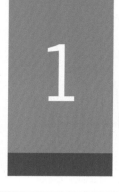

# 1 Introduction to Echocardiographic Principles

Jose A. Madrazo and Suzanne V. Arnold

## HIGH-YIELD CONCEPTS

- Pulsed-wave Doppler is RANGE specific but limited in the peak velocity it can measure.
- Continuous-wave Doppler is able to measure HIGH velocities but cannot localize the origin along its beam.
- M-mode has high TEMPORAL resolution but is limited by oblique imaging of structures of interest.

## KEY FORMULAS

- *Simplified Bernoulli Equation: $\Delta P(mmHg) = 4 \times V^2$ ($V = m/sec$)*
- LVOT area = $\pi \times$ (LVOT diameter in cm/2)$^2$
- Stroke volume = (LVOT area) $\times$ (LVOT TVI)
- QP/QS = (RVOT area) $\times$ (RVOT TVI)/(LVOT area) $\times$ (LVOT TVI)
- **Continuity principle for aortic valve area = (LVOT area) $\times$ (LVOT VTI)/(AoV VTI)**

- **Echocardiography uses sound waves to create images of the heart and other structures.**
  - Sound waves are mechanical vibrations described in terms of frequency or Hertz (Hz) = the number of cycles per second.
  - The frequency used by the ultrasound transducer affects image resolution and tissue penetration.
    - High frequency = high resolution image, low tissue penetration.
    - Low frequency = low resolution image, high tissue penetration.
  - Ultrasound refers to sound waves with 20 kHz or higher.
    - Adult echocardiography typically uses frequencies of 2 to 7 MHz.
  - Transthoracic echocardiography employs low-frequency transducers (2 to 4 MHz), which allows deeper penetration through the chest wall but at the expense of reduced resolution.

  - **Key Point:** *It is sometimes useful to decrease the transducer frequency in obese patients in order to improve image quality.*

  - Transesophageal echocardiography does not require deep tissue penetration and can use higher frequency transducers (3.5 to 7 MHz) to produce higher resolution images.

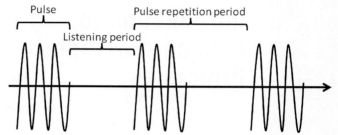

**Figure 1-1.** Description of ultrasound waves using standardized nomenclature.

- Piezoelectric elements are crystals that convert electrical energy into mechanical sound waves and vice versa. These crystals are in the transducer and their properties, number, and movement determine the characteristics of the images obtained.
- **Harmonic imaging:** Tissue and contrast bubbles not only reflect ultrasound at the transmitted frequency but also resonate at multiples of that frequency (harmonic frequencies). Harmonic imaging refers to setting the transducer to receive frequencies at multiples of the emitted frequency (e.g., Transmit at 3 MHz and receive at 6 MHz, the second harmonic). Harmonic imaging improves signal to noise ratio and the delineation of the endocardial border.
- **Mechanical index (MI):** A measure of the mechanical pressure exerted on tissues by the ultrasound waves. It is important to **lower the MI during contrast echocardiography** so as not to burst the contrast bubbles quickly.
- **Frame rate:** The number of still images displayed sequentially per unit of time. Multiple still images displayed sequentially lead to the perception of motion, thus higher frame rates lead to better temporal resolution but may sacrifice image quality and vice versa.

---

- **Key Point:** *Shallower imaging and narrower imaging sector can be easily adjusted to allow for higher frame rates and better temporal resolution.*

---

- **Pulse repetition period:** A pulse of ultrasound of a given frequency is sent by the transducer followed by a prespecified "listening period" before the transducer senses waves of the same frequency and generates an image. The duration of the pulse plus the time spent listening is referred to as the pulse repetition period. The longer this period is the deeper the images obtained (Fig. 1-1).

## Basic Imaging Modalities:

- **M-mode echocardiography:**
  - M-mode echocardiography depicts the structures along the path of a single line of the ultrasound beam. The still image of these structures is continuously updated over time on the 'x' axis. Thus, the structures along the line of the ultrasound beam are depicted as they change with time (Fig. 1-2).

---

- **Key Point:** *It may be useful to visualize the M-mode transducer as a virtual ice-pick with the structures along its path depicted on the screen and updated horizontally over time.*

---

- Because of its high sampling frequency (up to 1000 pulses per second), M-mode has excellent axial resolution and is useful in identifying the relative location of structures and measuring range of motion.
- **M-mode also has better temporal resolution than 2D imaging** and thus subtle abnormalities in motion and timing may be better appreciated with M-mode. For

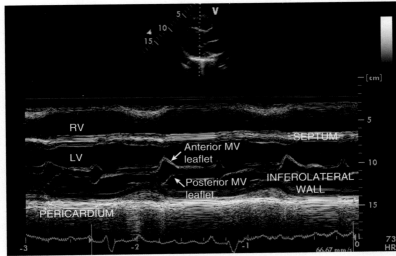

**Figure 1-2.** M-mode providing an "ice-pick" view of changes in cardiac structures seen in the parasternal long-axis view over time.

example systolic anterior motion of the mitral valve in HCM and right ventricular diastolic collapse in cardiac tamponade may be better appreciated by M-mode.

- **Two-dimensional echocardiography:**
  - The cardiac structures in the plane defined by the transducer position are depicted in two dimensions on the screen and the screen is updated continuously (see frame rate above), thus producing a "movie."
  - In adult echocardiography, structures closest to the transducer are displayed at the top of the screen, and the side of the ultrasound plane that corresponds to the **notch** on the transducer is on the **right** side of the screen.

  ---
  - **Key Point:** *It may be initially useful to imagine the transducer as a virtual blade with its plane in the same orientation as the notch on the transducer. The placement, rotation, and tilt of this "blade" will determine how you slice the heart and therefore the image obtained.*
  ---

  - Imaging the heart in multiple 2D planes allows for the reconstruction and visualization of all the parts of a 3D structure.
- **Three-dimensional echocardiography:**
  - Multiple 2D planes can be pieced together in order to recreate a 3D structure. Modern 3D echocardiography transducers accomplish this by imaging along a pyramidal ultrasound beam (instead of a knife, the beam is an inverted cone with the tip at the transducer).

## Doppler Principle and Applications:

- **Doppler effect:**
  - Proposed in 1842 by Austrian physicist Christian Doppler, it is the change in frequency of a wave received by an observer (the reflected frequency) relative to the source of the wave (originating frequency).

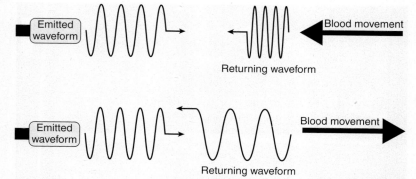

**Figure 1-3.** Diagram showing how the direction and speed of movement of an object changes the frequency of the reflected ultrasound wave (Doppler shift).

- When sound is emitted from a source at a given frequency and it is reflected from a static source the waves return at the same frequency emitted.
- However, when sound is reflected from a moving source the received frequency is shifted proportionally to the source's velocity.
  ○ If the object is moving toward the transducer, the resulting frequency is higher than the originating frequency and there is a "positive Doppler shift."
  ○ If the object is moving away from the transducer, the resulting frequency is lower than the originating frequency and there is a "negative Doppler shift" (Fig. 1-3).
- The angle at which the object is moving relative to the observer influences the magnitude of the Doppler shift—that is, the measured velocity of the blood is related to both the true velocity of the blood and the angle at which it is measured.
  ○ From a mathematical perspective, the Doppler shift is proportional to the cosine of the angle between the sound emitter and the moving object: $\text{velocity}_{\text{measured}} = \text{cosine of angle } (\Theta) \times \text{velocity}_{\text{true}}$ (Fig. 1-4).

- **Key Point:** *In order not to underestimate the velocity of a jet, it is important that the ultrasound beam is as parallel as possible to the direction of blood flow (i.e., cosine of zero degrees is one meaning measured velocity is equal to true velocity). This is accomplished by using multiple views, non-imaging transducers (i.e., Pedoff), and guidance by color Doppler.*

| | Blood flow (0) | Blood flow (30) | Blood flow (45) | Blood flow (60) | Blood flow (90) |
|---|---|---|---|---|---|
| Angle (Θ) | 0 | 30 | 45 | 60 | 90 |
| Cosine of Θ | 1 | 0.87 | 0.7 | 0.5 | 0 |
| Measured velocity | 5 m/s | 4.35 m/s | 3.5 m/s | 2.5 m/s | 0 m/s |

**Figure 1-4.** The effect of angle of insonation in measuring a jet with a true velocity of 5 m/s by Doppler echocardiography.

- **Pulsed-wave Doppler:**
  - In pulsed-wave (PW) Doppler, the transducer sends pulses of ultrasound at a given frequency and interrogates for Doppler shift at a specific site defined in a 2D image (**sample volume**).
  - **Pulse repetition frequency (PRF)** refers to the number of pulses in one second, and is therefore inversely proportional to pulse repetition period. A **low PRF is used to image deeper structures**.
  - The PRF determines the depth at which the Doppler shift is evaluated.
    - Lower PRF allows for longer "listening time" between the pulses and therefore interrogates at a deeper level and vice versa.
  - *Nyquist limit:* Named after Swedish-American engineer, Harry Nyquist, who discovered that the number of pulses per unit time is limited to twice the bandwidth of the channel. In practical terms, Nyquist limit = one-half PRF.
    - If the velocity of blood flow exceeds the Nyquist limit, the direction and velocity are inaccurately displayed and appear to change direction, a phenomenon termed **aliasing**.
  - PW is limited by the maximum velocity that can be measured, as the next pulse cannot be sent out before the signal is returned. The highest velocity that can be accurately measured is the Nyquist limit. Velocities greater than the Nyquist limit appear on the opposite side of the scale, aliasing (Fig. 1-5).

---

- **Key Point:** *PW allows for determination of flow velocity at a specific point (sample volume) but is limited to measuring only lower velocities because of aliasing.*

---

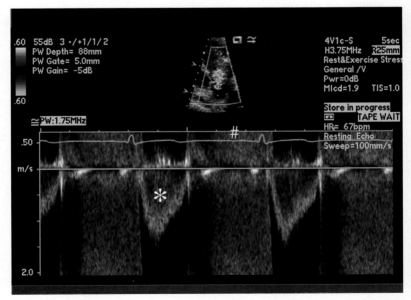

**Figure 1-5.** A spectral display from pulsed-wave Doppler in the LVOT shows aliasing of the high velocity aortic regurgitant jet (#). Lower velocity flow in systole does not alias (*).

---

- **Key Point:** *Imaging shallower structures allows for use of a higher PRF and therefore higher Nyquist limit. Use views that minimize the distance to the jet of interest if aliasing is a problem.*

---

- **Continuous-wave Doppler:**
  - In continuous-wave (CW) Doppler, the transducer has some crystals dedicated to constantly emitting ultrasound while other crystals continuously "listen" for a shift in frequency.
  - Because the ultrasound beam is continuous, CW is not limited by PRF in the velocities it detects (i.e., there is no aliasing). Hence, **CW can interrogate high velocity flows**.
  - Since the shift occurs anywhere along the path of the beam, **CW cannot localize the position along that beam where the highest velocity occurs** (Table 1-1).

---

  - **Key Point:** *CW allows for the determination of the* highest *flow velocity* anywhere *along the ultrasound beam but cannot localize the point of maximal velocity. It is not range-specific.*

---

  - A *Pedoff* probe is a specialized non-imaging CW transducer that contains two elements—one element is always transmitting while the other is always receiving. It provides very accurate CW Doppler data and, due to its very small size, is useful for assessing peak velocities from high parasternal and suprasternal views and in patients with a challenging body habitus.
- **High pulse repetition frequency (HPRF) pulsed Doppler:**
  - Attempts to overcome the limitations of CW in depth ambiguity and PW in aliasing.
  - HPRF is a variant of PW, where one or more new pulses are sent out before the echo from the first is received. This shortens the PRF and thereby increases the Nyquist limit and results in multiple sample volumes.
  - HPRF increases the accuracy of high velocity measurements at the cost of depth ambiguity, as it is unknown which sampling volume is the site of the highest velocity. Thus it results in "partial depth ambiguity."

| **TABLE 1-1** | Characteristics of the Different Doppler Modes | | |
|---|---|---|---|
| | **Advantages** | **Disadvantages** | **Common uses** |
| **CW** | Measures high velocity flows | Cannot determine site of high velocity | Peak and mean aortic and mitral stenosis gradients, regurgitation jets |
| **PW** | Measures velocity at a specific location | Cannot assess high velocities | Ventricular outflow tract, mitral valve inflow, pulmonary veins |
| **HPRF** | Increased Nyquist limit | Cannot tell which sampling volume contains the high velocity | Left ventricular outflow obstruction |

• **Key Point:** *HPRF is ideal for trying to determine where along a beam the high velocity occurs and is most often used in the setting of a dynamic left ventricular outflow tract (LVOT) obstruction (i.e., hypertrophic cardiomyopathy).*

• **Color Doppler:**
  • Color Doppler is a variation of PW in which multiple sample volumes in a 2D plane are interrogated simultaneously. Each sample's velocity is assigned a color according to a prespecified scheme and superimposed on the underlying 2D image (Fig. 1-6).
  • By convention, most echocardiography labs display flow going away from the transducer as blue and flow toward as red *(Blue-Away, Red-Toward)*.
  • Higher velocity flow has progressively lighter shades of the same color until the Nyquist limit is reached at which point aliasing occurs and the color changes to the opposite one (i.e., blue to red or red to blue).
  • In order to highlight turbulence, many machines add a third color (such as green or yellow) to areas with a wide variability of flow velocities and directions. This feature can be turned off if needed to make the direction of blood flow more explicit.
  • Color Doppler allows for a quick visual assessment of location, velocity, and turbulence of blood flow in a given region.

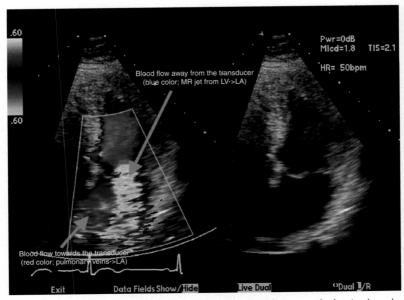

**Figure 1-6.** Color Doppler of blood flow in the LA and LV during systole showing how the direction and velocity of flow is represented.

- **Tissue Doppler imaging (TDI):**
  - TDI is a variation of PW Doppler that uses the principles of Doppler imaging to assess myocardial tissue velocity (typically <20 cm/s), which is much lower than blood flow velocity (measured in m/s).
  - In conventional PW, the lower velocities generated by cardiac tissue are filtered out to focus on the higher velocities from moving blood cells. This filter is inactived during TDI, allowing measurement of the higher amplitude lower velocity signals of tissue motion.

  - **Key Point:** *TDI is typically used in the assessment of diastolic function, right ventricular function, and myocardial strain.*

## Useful Hemodynamic Principles and Applications:

- **Stroke volume and other flow volumes:**
  - The volume of blood traveling through an orifice can be estimated by multiplying the area through which the blood travels by the velocity of blood flow through that orifice for the duration of the time period of assessment (Fig. 1-7).
  - Stroke volume (SV) is defined as the volume of blood ejected from the LV per beat. A simple determination of stroke volume can be made by measuring forward flow velocity in the LVOT and calculating the area of the LVOT.
  - First, the LVOT cross-sectional area is determined by direct measurement of the LVOT diameter. Assuming the LVOT is circular, the area is calculated by the following formula:
    - LVOT area in $cm^2 = \pi \times$ (LVOT diameter in cm/2)$^2$.

    - **Key Point:** *LVOT diameter is usually best measured in the parasternal long-axis view in early to mid-systole using a magnified view.*

  - If flow across an orifice is constant (like in a garden hose), then multiplying the velocity of the flow (cm/s) by the orifice area (cm$^2$) calculates the flow rate (cm$^3$/s). The flow rate multiplied by the ejection time calculates the volume of flow. However, blood pumped by the heart is not only pulsatile, but the velocity of flow also varies throughout the systolic ejection period. In order to accurately determine the volume of blood pumped per beat, we must use a sum of the velocities over the systolic ejection period in order to create an average.

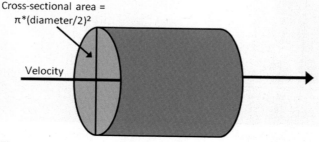

Cross-sectional area =
$\pi$*(diameter/2)$^2$

Velocity

**Figure 1-7.** Diagram illustrating the assumption that blood flow through a cylinder approximates flow through a cardiac orifice.

- By integrating the flow velocity over time we obtain the velocity time integral (VTI), a measure of distance (cm); also termed stroke distance.
  - From a conceptual point of view the systolic LVOT VTI represents the distance a single blood cell would travel during one beat in a cylinder with a cross-sectional area equal to the LVOT.
  - The VTI is measured by obtaining a PW measurement at the LVOT and then tracing it on the screen. The computer calculates the area under the curve and reads out the VTI.

  > • Key Point: *LVOT VTI is best obtained from the apical five- or apical long-axis views.*

- LVOT area (cm$^2$) multiplied by stroke distance (cm/beat) yields SV (cm$^3$/beat or mL/beat).
  - **SV = (LVOT TVI) × (LVOT area)**
- Taking this concept further, SV can then be multiplied by heart rate to calculate cardiac output (CO), which divided by body surface area (BSA) equals cardiac index (CI; divide by 1,000 to convert to mL to L).
  - **CO (L/min) = SV (mL/beat)/1000 × heart rate (beats/min)**
  - **CI (L/min/m$^2$) = CO (L/min)/BSA (m$^2$)**
- **The above concept may be applied to any orifice to measure blood flow.**
- For example, this principle can be used to determine mitral regurgitation severity by a "volumetric method." Calculate how much blood flows into the left ventricle (LV) using (MV annulus area × diastolic VTI **at that level**) and comparing it to SV (as calculated above) allows for determination of the volume of blood that regurgitates back into the left atrium (LA) during systole (LV inflow – LV outflow volume), known as the regurgitant volume. This will be discussed further in future chapters.
- Another application of this principle is to quantify a right to left shunt. This is done by comparing pulmonary flow (Qp) to systemic flow (Qs), where the ratio of pulmonary to systemic flow (Qp/Qs ratio) is considered elevated if >1.5. Qs is determined by the above SV calculation, and Qp is similarly calculated by multiplying the area of the right ventricular outflow tract (RVOT) by the RVOT systolic VTI.
  - **Qp/Qs = (RVOT area) × (RVOT VTI)/(LVOT area) × (LVOT VTI)**

  > • Key Point: *RVOT diameter and VTI are usually best obtained in the parasternal short-axis view at the level of the aortic valve. Alternatively, the proximal pulmonary artery (PA) diameter and PW VTI at the PA may be used.*

- **Bernoulli principle and estimation of pressure in cardiac chambers:**
  - The Bernoulli principle is a derivation of the Law of Conservation of Energy. Applied to echocardiography, if blood flow across a valve or orifice is viewed as fluid flowing through a cylinder of varying diameters, the energy of the fluid must be conserved at all points in the cylinder.
  - The main biologically relevant variables in this system are pressure and velocity of blood; other components such as flow acceleration, viscous friction, and gravitational energy are omitted for simplification.
    - Pressure Energy$_1$ (P$_1$) + Kinetic Energy$_1$ = Pressure Energy$_2$ (P$_2$) + Kinetic Energy$_2$
    - Kinetic energy of blood is calculated by the formula: $\frac{1}{2}\rho \times V^2$, where $\rho$ is the mass density of blood and $\frac{1}{2}\rho$ is roughly 4.
    - $P_1 + 4 \times V_1^2 = P_2 + 4 \times V_2^2$, or
    - $P_1 - P_2 \, (\Delta P) = 4 \times V_1^2 - 4 \times V_2^2$

- Since the velocity proximal to a fixed orifice ($V_2$) is usually much lower than the peak velocity across it, $V_2$ does not contribute significantly and can usually be ignored.
- **Simplified Bernoulli Equation:** $\Delta P(mmHg) = 4 \times V^2$
  - Using the Simplified Bernoulli Equation, we can estimate the pressure gradient across an orifice between two cardiac chambers. If the pressure in one chamber is known (or estimated), then the pressure in the adjacent chamber can be calculated by determining the pressure difference between the two chambers.
  - The most common application of this principle is the estimation of pulmonary artery systolic pressure (PASP). In the absence of RVOT obstruction or pulmonic valve stenosis, PASP equals RV systolic pressure (RVSP). Peak tricuspid regurgitation (TR) velocity reflects the difference between RVSP and RA pressure.
    - $4 \times (\text{peak TR velocity})^2 = \text{RVSP} - \text{RA pressure}$
    - $\text{RVSP} = 4 \times (\text{peak TR velocity})^2 + \text{RA pressure}$
- RA pressure is estimated clinically by measuring jugular venous pressure (JVP) or by echocardiography by measuring the inferior vena cava (IVC) diameter (see Chapter 5).
- **Continuity principle:**
  - The continuity principle is an extension of the Law of Conservation of Mass. In incompressible fluid dynamics, the flow rate varies according to the cross-sectional area in order for the volume (mass) to be preserved. Simply stated in echocardiography, the volume of blood going in must equal that going out (Fig. 1-8).
  - As explained above, the product of VTI and the cross-sectional area where the VTI is measured, can measure volume.
  - Therefore by **continuity principle (or continuity equation):**
    - $(A_1) \times (VTI_1) = (A_2) \times (VTI_2)$
  - The continuity equation is commonly applied to the measurement of aortic valve area (AVA) in patients with aortic valve (AoV) stenosis (AS). Flow velocity will be greatest at the narrowest portion (the stenotic AoV valve in the case of AS) and can be determined by CW Doppler. Therefore AVA can be calculated by measuring LVOT diameter, PW Doppler at LVOT, and CW Doppler across the AoV.
    - $(AVA) \times (\text{VTI from AoV CW}) = (\text{LVOT area}) \times (\text{VTI from PW at LVOT})$, or
    - $\text{AVA} = (\text{LVOT area}) \times (\text{LVOT VTI})/(\text{AoV VTI})$

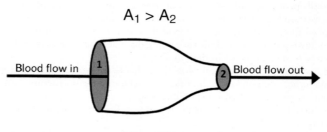

$$A_1 > A_2$$

Blood flow in 1      2 Blood flow out →

$$V_1 < V_2$$

**Figure 1-8.** Diagram illustrating the continuity principle which states that the product of the cross-sectional area and velocity time integral are the same for blood entering and leaving the heart.

Table 1-2 summarizes the application of Doppler echocardiography to measure cardiac hemodynamic indices.

| TABLE 1-2 | Assessing Cardiac Hemodynamic Indices by Echocardiography | |
| --- | --- | --- |
| Hemodynamic | Parameters needed | Calculation |
| **Stroke volume** | LVOT VTI, LVOT diameter | $SV = \pi \times (\text{LVOT diameter}/2)^2 \times (\text{LVOT VTI})$ |
| **Cardiac output** | LVOT VTI, LVOT diameter, heart rate | $CO = \pi \times (\text{LVOT diameter}/2)^2 \times (\text{LVOT VTI}) \times HR$ |
| **RA pressure/CVP** | IVC diameter (see Chapter 5) | IVC ≤ 2.1 cm with respiratory variation >50% = 0–5 mmHg<br>IVC > 2.1 cm with respiratory variation <50% = 10–20 mmHg<br>IVC changes not fitting the above are categorized by an intermediate RA pressure value of 5–10 mmHg. |
| **PASP** | TR jet, IVC diameter | $4 \times (\text{peak TR jet})^2$ + estimated RAP |
| **LVEDP**[a] | E/e′ (see Chapter 4) | • <5 = normal LVEDP<br>• >15 = elevated LVEDP |

[a]LVEDP, Left Ventricular End Diastolic Pressure.

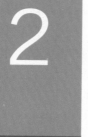

# 2 The Comprehensive Transthoracic Echocardiographic Examination

Pei-Hsiu Huang

## GETTING STARTED

A quality echocardiogram study starts with the setup (Fig. 2-1).

### Patient Positioning

The low-powered ultrasound beam cannot image the entire heart clearly in its natural position behind the sternum.

*Helpful Tips:*
- Use the left lateral decubitus position to shift the heart laterally.
- Place a wedge or pillow to support the patient on their left side.
- Raise the left arm above the head to spread the intercostal spaces.

**Patient comfort is key!**

### Sonographer Positioning

Get comfortable to prevent frequent breaks or a hastily performed examination. The examination can be performed from either side of the patient.

*Helpful Tips:*
- The examination table height should allow the sonographer's elbow to rest comfortably with a slight arm bend.
- Position the patient so the examination can be performed without leaning.

### Handling the Transducer

*Helpful Tips:*
- The transducer should rest between thumb and index and middle fingers (much like throwing a dart).
- Move the fingers to the tip of the transducer.
- Stabilize the transducer against the patient's chest using the little finger.
- Note the position of the transducer notch (N) to orient the cardiac views.

### Machine Setup

Move the machine beyond the head of the bed allowing space to sit at the level of the patient's chest. Make sure to record the following information for each examination:

| | |
|---|---|
| *Patient identification* | **Full name**<br>**Date of birth**<br>**Identification number** |
| *Vitals* | **Height/weight** (used for indexing measurements)<br>**Blood pressure** (evaluating hemodynamic significance) |

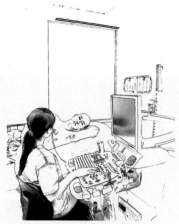

**Figure 2-1.** Echocardiogram setup.

| Additional Imaging Considerations | |
|---|---|
| **Acoustic Windows**<br>The optimal acoustic window allows acquisition of bright and clear images. Poor image quality will affect the accuracy of 2D measurements and Doppler quality. | • Acquire the "big picture" first<br>• Move the transducer along and between the intercostal spaces<br>• **Keep the transducer movements small** |
| **Respiration**<br>Heart position changes with respiration. | • Acquire most **parasternal** and **apical** views at held **end-expiration**<br>• Acquire the **apical two-chamber** and **subcostal** views at held **end-inspiration** |
| **Transducer Pressure**<br>Firm pressure is necessary for good transducer contact. However, applying too much pressure, especially on pain sensitive bony surfaces, will cause the patient pain! | • When imaging through areas of increased subcutaneous tissue (e.g., adipose tissue or under breasts), **applying increased pressure** often improves the image quality<br>• Slightly reduce pressure, once a good quality image is found<br>• Release the transducer pressure when switching intercostal spaces |
| **Ultrasound Gel**<br>A medium used to conduct sound waves between the patient and the ultrasound transducer | • Use plenty of gel!<br>• Reapply when the gel on the patient spreads to a thin layer |

## ADJUSTING THE IMAGE

### 2D Gain

The intracardiac blood pool should be as dark as possible without losing definition of the cardiac structures (Fig. 2-2).

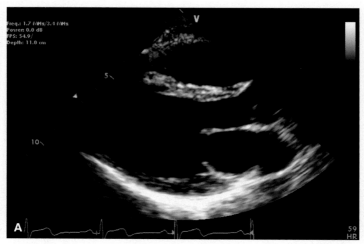

**Figure 2-2A.** Optimum gain.

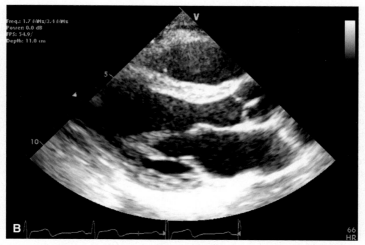

**Figure 2-2B.** Over-gained.

## IMAGE DEPTH

The depth should be set to extend approximately 1 to 2 cm beyond the cardiac boundary most distant from the transducer to ensure that none of the structures are cut off (Fig. 2-3).

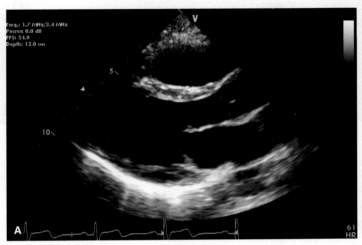

Figure 2-3A. Optimum depth.

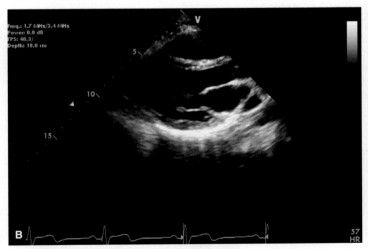

Figure 2-3B. Too deep.

*Note:* Some laboratories use standard default depths to facilitate comparison of serial examinations. In this case, acquire images at the default depth as well as at the appropriate depth.

## Color Doppler

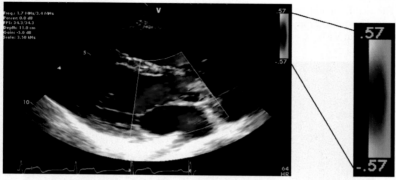

Figure 2-4. Color Doppler sampling region with Nyquist limit (inset).

Adjust the color Doppler sampling region to include only the structures of interest in order to avoid decreases in temporal resolution and color quality. Keep the default Nyquist limit at 50–60 cm/s (Fig. 2-4).

## Color Gain

This can be calibrated by moving the color box into the extracardiac space and increasing Doppler gain until there is visible noise. Slowly decrease gain until the noise first disappears.

## Frequency

Start imaging with the transducer set at 1.7/3.4 MHz (transmitted/received; second harmonic imaging) (Fig. 2-5). Select a higher (for near-field imaging) or lower (for deeper penetration) frequency to optimize the image quality.

**Freq.: 1.7 MHz/3.4 MHz**
**Power: 0.0 dB**
**FPS: 54.9**
**Depth: 12.0 cm**

Figure 2-5. Transducer setting.

## Focus

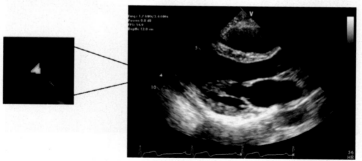

Figure 2-6. The focus of the ultrasound beam is shown by the arrow (inset).

Try adjusting the ultrasound focus if an unclear image or artifact is encountered (Fig. 2-6).

## Pulsed-wave Doppler Sample Volume Sizes

Inflow/outflow: 3 to 4 mm
Venous flow: 5 to 7 mm
Tissue or annular velocities: 5 to 7 mm

An inappropriate sample size may contaminate the Doppler acquisition and nullify spectral Doppler's greatest advantage of range specificity.

## Spectral Gain

The background should be dark and the signal bright to ensure it is not under-gained. Over-gained images may result in over-estimation of blood flow velocities. Measurements should be taken of the modal velocities (bright envelope) and not the spectral broadening ("feathery spray") especially seen in over-gained or poor quality Doppler (Fig. 2-7).

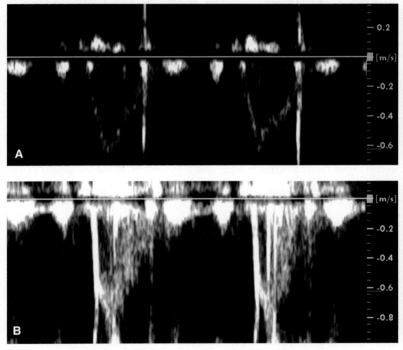

Figure 2-7. (A) Pulsed-wave Doppler with appropriate gain and (B) over-gained.

## Sweep Speed

Generally set at 50 mm/s for M-mode and spectral Doppler with normal heart rates. Set the sweep speed at 100 mm/s to get measurements at a high temporal resolution (Fig. 2-8).

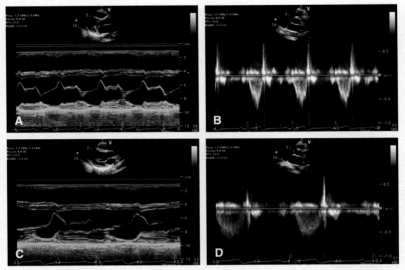

**Figure 2-8.** PLAX view with M-mode through the mitral valve leaflets and PSAX view with spectral Doppler of the RVOT with sweep speed at 50 mm/s **(A, B)** and 100 mm/s **(C, D)**.

## PARASTERNAL LONG AXIS (PLAX)

See Figure 2-9.

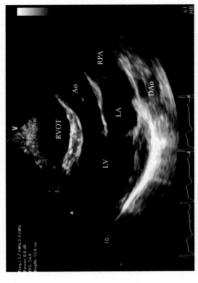

*Obtaining the Image:*

- At the third or fourth intercostal space, point the notch toward the patient's right shoulder.
- Keep the transducer close to but not on the sternum.
- Move the transducer superiorly (High PLAX) to measure aortic root dimensions.

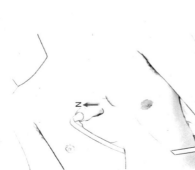

Figure 2-9. Parasternal long-axis (PLAX) view. *N,* transducer notch.

### 2D Examination

*Structures*

- *Chambers:* LA, LV, LVOT, RVOT, Ao, DAo, RPA
- *Valves:* MV, AoV

*Key Features*

- Coaptation of the anterior and posterior MV leaflets.
- Coaptation of the AoV leaflets. The right coronary cusp is closest to the RVOT with either the non or left cusp opposite it.
- LV cavity is maximized (imaging between papillary muscles).

### Doppler Examination

*Color Doppler*

- MV and AoV: Color box should include the IVS, AoV, and MV
- Especially useful in this view for identifying eccentric regurgitant jets, ventricular septal defects and assessing aortic regurgitation (AR) severity

### M-mode Examination

*Chambers*

- Mid-ventricle to include the antero-septum and inferolateral walls

*Valves*

- MV and AoV structure and leaflet motion

# RIGHT VENTRICULAR INFLOW TRACT

See Figure 2-10.

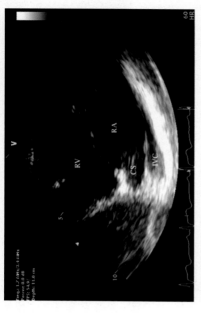

*Obtaining the Image:*
- From the PLAX view tilt the transducer tail toward the left shoulder.
- The imaging plane will slowly move anteriorly until the TV is in view.

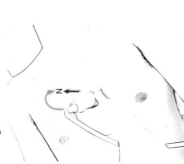

Figure 2-10. Right ventricular inflow tract (RVIT) view. *N*, transducer notch.

## 2D Examination

*Structures*
- *Chambers:* RA, RV, IVC, CS
- *Valves:* TV

*Key Features*
- This is the only view the posterior TV leaflet is seen.
- Coaptation of the TV leaflets.

## Doppler Examination

*Color Doppler*
- TV: Color box should include the RA, TV, and RV

*Spectral Doppler*
- CW: Place the cursor through the vena contracta of the TV regurgitant jet (or the valve leaflet coaptation point if the vena contracta is not visualized).

## Troubleshooting

The transducer tilt for this view is often directed toward a rib. Open the acoustic window by:
- Sliding the transducer laterally away from the right ventricle
- Moving to a lower intercostal space if the image continues to be difficult to obtain

# PARASTERNAL SHORT AXIS (PSAX)

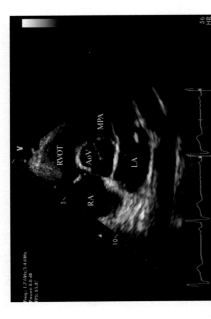

*Obtaining the image:*

- From the PLAX view, rotate the transducer clockwise 90° (red arrow)
- Tilt the transducer tail slightly toward the right shoulder for more apical views and away from the right shoulder for basal views (blue arrows)

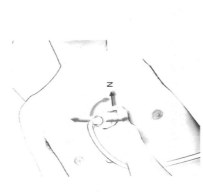

Figure 2-11. Parasternal short-axis (PSAX) view. *N,* transducer notch.

## 2D Examination (Aortic Valve Level)

See Figure 2-11.

*Structures*
- *Chambers:* LA, RA, RV/RVOT, MPA
- *Valves:* AoV, TV, PV

*Key Features*
- The three leaflets of the AoV with a circular aortic root.

## Doppler Examination (Aortic Valve Level)

*Color Doppler*
- AoV: Size color box to include the AoV
- PV: Color box should include the RVOT, PV, and MPA
- TV: Color box should include the RA, TV, and interatrial septum

*Spectral Doppler*
- PW: PV (place sample volume in the RVOT, 1 cm proximal to PV)
- CW: Place cursor through the vena contracta of the TV or PV regurgitant jet, or the valve leaflet coaptation point.

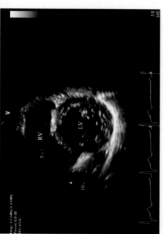

Figure 2-12. 2D examination, mitral valve level.

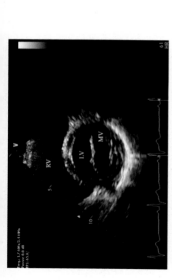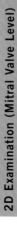

Figure 2-13. 2D examination, papillary muscle level.

## 2D Examination (Mitral Valve Level)

See Figure 2-12.

*Structures*
- *Chambers:* LV, RV
- *Valves:* MV

*Key Features*
- Anterior and posterior MV leaflets with the coaptation point at the center of the ventricle.

Tip: If the valve appears to open medially, rotate the transducer clockwise for a more complete view; if it opens laterally, rotate counterclockwise.

## Doppler Examination (Mitral Valve Level)

*Color Doppler*
- MV: Color box should include the MV

*Spectral Doppler*
- Generally not useful in this view

## 2D Examination (Papillary Muscle Level)

See Figure 2-13.

*Structures*
- *Chambers:* LV, RV

*Key Features*
- Circular shape of the LV
- Anterolateral and posteromedial papillary muscles

## Doppler Examination (Papillary Muscle Level)

Color and spectral Doppler are not generally useful in this view.

## Troubleshooting (PSAX)

**Rib artifacts** are common and can be minimized by sliding the transducer away from the rib shadowing the ventricle.

# APICAL FOUR-CHAMBER (A4C)

See Figure 2-14.

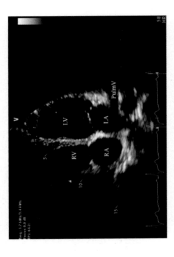

*Obtaining the Image:*
- This view is generally found near (not actually over) the point of maximum impulse.
- Angle the transducer tail away from the patient's right shoulder.

## 2D Examination

*Structures*
- Chambers: LA, RA, LV (inferoseptal and anterolateral walls), RV, PulmV
- Valves: MV, TV

*Key Features*
- Entire length of the LV is visualized.
- Well-defined LV endocardium in all segments.
- Coaptation of the MV and TV (septal and anterior) leaflets.
- RV free wall and TV annulus motion.

## Doppler Examination

*Color Doppler*
- MV: Color box should include LA, MV, LV inflow
- TV: Color box should include RA, TV, RV, interatrial septum, IVS

*Spectral Doppler*
- PW: MV (place sample volume at leaflet tips; for volumetric calculations place sample at mitral annulus level), PulmV
- CW: Place cursor through the vena contracta of regurgitant jet or MV and TV leaflet coaptation point
- TD: Septal and lateral MV annuli; lateral TV annulus

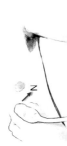

Figure 2-14. Apical four-chamber (A4C) view. *N,* transducer notch.

## Troubleshooting

*Common Problems:*
- Ventricles visualized, but not the atria: Tilt the transducer up or down
- MV/TV coaptation or LV/RV cut-off: Rotate transducer clockwise or counterclockwise
- Apex not centered: Move transducer medially or laterally

*Note:* The location of the optimal acoustic window also varies depending on how much the patient is rolled onto their left side (i.e., if the patient is supine the apical window will be more medial).

## APICAL FIVE-CHAMBER (A5C)

See Figure 2-15.

*Obtaining the Image:*
- From the A4C view, tilt the transducer tail toward the patient's left hip (red arrow)

  *Note:* the aortic valve plane lies only a few degrees anterior to the A4C plane.

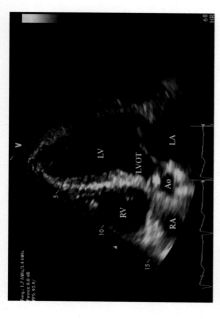

**Figure 2-15.** Apical five-chamber (A5C) view. *N,* transducer notch.

### 2D Examination

*Structures*
- *Chambers:* LA, RA, LV, LVOT, RV, Ao
- *Valves:* MV, TV, AoV

*Key Features*
- Similar to A4C with additional visualization of the LVOT, AoV, and Ao root.

### Doppler Examination

*Color Doppler*
- Color box should include the AoV

*Spectral Doppler*
- PW: LVOT (place the sample volume ~1 cm proximal to the AV
- CW: Place cursor through the vena contracta of the AoV regurgitant jet, or the valve leaflet coaptation point to evaluate aortic stenosis.

## APICAL TWO-CHAMBER (A2C)
See Figure 2-16.

### 2D Examination

*Structures*
- *Chambers:* LA, LV (anterior and inferior walls)
- *Valves:* MV

*Key Features*
- Entire length of the LV with well-defined endocardial segments.
- Coaptation of the MV leaflets.
- Occasionally, the LAA and CS can be visualized.

*Obtaining the Image:*
- From the A4C view, rotate the transducer roughly 30° counterclockwise (red arrow).

*Be careful not to foreshorten the LV by moving the transducer medially.*

### Doppler Examination

*Color Doppler*
- MV: Color box should include the LA, MV, and LV inflow

*Spectral Doppler*
- PW: Generally, place the sample volume at MV leaflet tips; for volumetric calculations, place the sample volume at the mitral annulus level
- CW: MV leaflet coaptation point

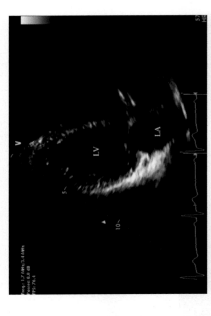

**Figure 2-16.** Apical two-chamber (A2C) view. *N*, transducer notch.

### Troubleshooting

This view is difficult to obtain because of two common problems:
- The transducer slips as you rotate
- The transducer is not at the apex

Tip: Anchor the transducer with one hand and rotate it with the other

25

# APICAL LONG AXIS (APLAX)

See Figure 2-17.

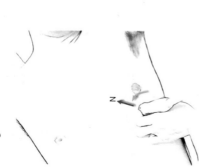

*Obtaining the Image:*
* From the A2C view, rotate the transducer roughly 30° counter-clockwise (red arrow).

*Be careful not to fore-shorten the LV by moving the transducer medially.*

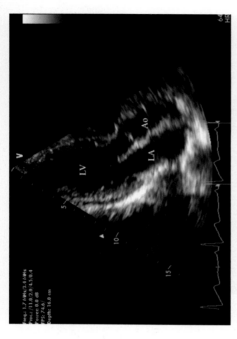

**Figure 2-17.** Apical long-axis (APLAX) view. *N*, transducer notch.

## 2D Examination

*Structures*
* *Chambers:* LA, LV (anteroseptal and inferolateral walls), Ao
* *Valves:* MV, AoV

*Key Features*
* Coaptation of the MV and AoV leaflets.

## Doppler Examination

*Color Doppler*
* MV and AoV: Color box should include the IVS, AoV, and MV

*Spectral Doppler*
* PW: LVOT, MV inflow
* CW: MV for regurgitation and AoV for aortic stenosis

## SUBCOSTAL CORONAL
See Figure 2-18.

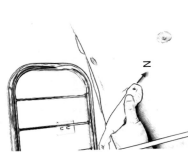

*Obtaining the Image:*
- With the patient lying supine, apply firm pressure at a 45° angle two finger-widths below the xiphoid process
- Aim the transducer up toward the patient's left shoulder

## 2D Examination

*Structures*
- *Chambers*: LA, RA, LV, RV
- *Valves*: MV, TV

*Key Features*
- LV function.
- Pericardial effusion and tamponade physiology if effusion present.
- Look for interatrial septal defects.

## Doppler Examination

*Color Doppler*
- MV: Color box should include the LA and MV
- TV: Color box should include the RA and TV
- Interatrial septum

*Spectral Doppler*
- CW: Through TV coaptation or vena contracta of regurgitant jet

## Troubleshooting

- Utilize the liver's low acoustic impedance by imaging slightly to the right of the xiphoid process
- Image at end-inspiration
- Relax the abdominal muscles by bending the patient's knees
- Decrease the transducer frequency to increase the depth of ultrasound penetration

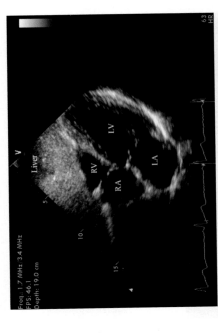

Freq. 1.7 MHz; 3.4 MHz
FPS: 46.1
Depth: 19.0 cm

63
HR

Figure 2-18. Subcostal coronal view. *N*, transducer notch.

# SUBCOSTAL SAGITTAL

See Figure 2-19.

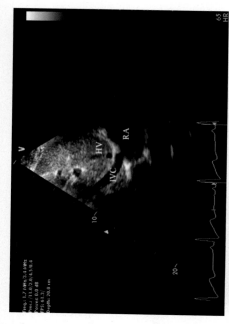

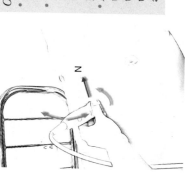

Figure 2-19. Subcostal sagittal view. *N*, transducer notch.

*Obtaining the Image:*
- Angle the transducer perpendicular to the patient.
- From the coronal view, rotate the transducer counterclockwise until the notch is toward the patient's head.
- A slight tilt of the transducer tail to the patient's left brings the IVC into view, tilting to the patient's right brings the abdominal aorta into view.

## 2D Examination

*Structures*
- Chambers: RA, IVC, hepatic vein, DAo (not shown).

*Key Features*
- IVC size and change with respiration (may require "sniff" maneuver if there is no significant change in size with normal breathing).

## Doppler Examination

*Color Doppler*
- IVC and hepatic vein
- DAo for turbulent flow

*Spectral Doppler*
- PW: Hepatic vein and DAo

## SUPRASTERNAL NOTCH (SSN) See Figure 2-20.

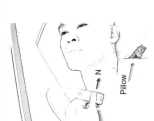

*Obtaining the Image:*
- Move the pillow under the shoulder blades, extending the patient's neck
- The transducer is placed above the suprasternal notch
- The transducer notch points to the patient's head with the transducer tail also angled slightly in this direction

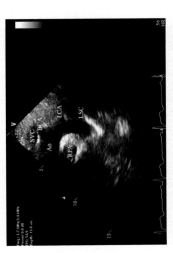

**Figure 2-20.** Suprasternal notch (SSN) view. *N,* transducer notch.

## 2D Examination

*Structures*
- *Chambers:* LA, aortic arch, brachiocephalic artery (BCA), left common carotid artery (LCA), left subclavian artery (LSC), and right pulmonary artery (RPA)

*Key Features*
- Look for anatomic abnormalities to suggest an aortic dissection, aortic coarctation, or patent ductus arteriosis.

## Doppler Examination

*Color Doppler*
- Arch vessels: Color box should include all of the arch vessels.

*Spectral Doppler*
- PW sampling of the proximal DAo (holodiastolic flow reversal seen in moderate to severe AR) or any areas of turbulence.
- CW of AoV for aortic valve jet.

## Tips for Technically Difficult Studies

*Patients with Hyperinflated Lungs*
The heart lies lower in the thoracic cavity in patients with longstanding pulmonary disease.
* Lower than normal parasternal windows should be attempted. It is not uncommon to obtain the best parasternal orientation from the subcostal view.
* Have the patient lie flat.
* Transducer orientation is the same and all axis views are often attainable.

*Obesity*
* Reduce transducer frequency for deeper penetration.
* Increase transducer pressure slightly for better tissue compression.
* Optimize width and depth.
* Decrease frame rates.

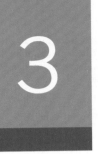

# 3

# The Role of Contrast in Echocardiography

Stephanie N. Johnson and Majesh Makan

## KEY POINTS FOR CONTRAST OPTIMIZATION

- Mechanical index (MI) <0.5
- Optimize time gain compensation and overall gain settings
- Minimize near-field gain
- Generally have focus point at the base of the heart
- Optimize probe position for non-foreshortened views
- Doppler enhancement measuring the modal/darkest envelope
- Correct timing and dose of contrast requires good communication between sonographer and nurse

## INDICATIONS

- Reduced image quality with ≥2 wall segments not visualized
- Increase the accuracy of ventricular volume measurement
- Stress testing for enhanced endocardial edge detection
- Doppler signal enhancement
- Evaluation for LV thrombus, LV aneurysm
- Intracardiac masses

## CONTRAINDICATIONS

- Pregnant or lactating women
- Patients who have known allergic reaction to Perflutren (Octafluropropane gas)
- Right-to-left, bi-directional or transient right-to-left cardiac shunts
- Sensitivity to blood, blood products, or albumin (Optison™ only)

## GENERAL PRINCIPLES

Using contrast while performing an echocardiogram can play a vital role and provide additional information in the patient's diagnosis and management. Contrast consists of microbubbles that when mixed with red blood cells in the cardiac chambers increase the scatter of the ultrasonic signal, therefore enhancing the blood–tissue interface. Optison™ is a Perfluoropropane-filled shell derived from human serum albumin, whereas Definity™ is a Perfluoropropane lipid–coated microbubble that has to be agitated before use. The FDA has approved contrast for left ventricular (LV) opacification and enhancement of endocardial border definition.

## Contrast Should be Given to Patient When:

- **Reduced image quality:** Two or more wall segments cannot be visualized in any one view.
- **Doppler signal enhancement**
  - For valvular stenosis and regurgitation
  - The best Doppler signal is obtained at the beginning of contrast administration. This helps avoid "blooming" artifact and overestimation of the Doppler signal
  - Measure only the modal envelope (Fig. 3-1)
- **Rule out LV apical pathology:** LV thrombus, aneurysm, pseudoaneurysm, apical hypertrophy, non-compaction (Fig. 3-2)

> - **Key Point:** *Move focus point transiently from the base of the heart to the apex to evaluate the LV apex for pathology.*

- **Assess regional wall motion abnormalities**
- **Exercise/pharmologic stress testing**
  - Ensures visualization of all myocardial segments
- **Increase accuracy of ejection fraction and LV volume calculations** (Fig. 3-3)
- **ICU and ER settings**
  - ICU patients are usually technically difficult to image due to mechanical ventilation, chest tubes, bandages, presence of lung disease, and inability for patients to be repositioned.
  - Most patients are imaged supine rather than in the left lateral position.
  - Using contrast in the ER is helpful when patients come in with chest pain to provide complete analysis of all myocardial segments for regional wall motion abnormalities.

> - **Key Point:** *Even though IV contrast may help with endocardial definition it does not reduce image foreshortening secondary to non-optimal probe or patient positioning. Try to optimize the image **prior** to contrast administration.*

- **Identifying intracardiac masses**
  - Thrombus does not enhance and is outlined as a "black" mass with contrast enhancement of the cardiac chambers.
  - Tumors within the cardiac chambers can similarly be outlined by contrast.
  - The use of contrast increases the sensitivity of detection of intracardiac masses and also helps in differentiating these from normal structures (e.g., LV trabeculation) (Fig. 3-4).

## PREPARING DEFINITY™ (LANTHEUS MEDICAL IMAGING) CONTRAST

- Definity™ has to be agitated in the vial mixer. Do not use unless it has completed the cycle. It is a clear liquid, which turns milky after activation.
- Draw 1.5 mL of Definity™ with a vented spike and dilute in 8.5 mL of saline.
- Turn MI down <0.5 to achieve maximum left ventricular opacification.
- Change gain settings to optimize endocardial border detection.

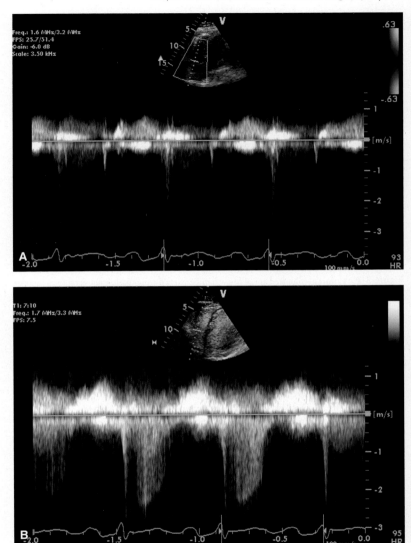

**Figure 3-1. A:** No measurable envelope is seen on spectral Doppler in patient with trace TR. **B:** After contrast enhancement a clear TR Doppler envelope can be accurately measured.

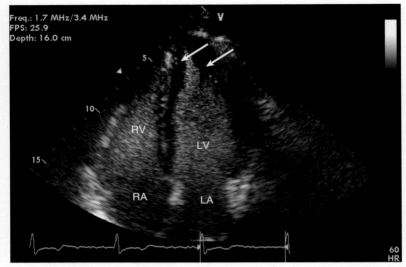

**Figure 3-2.** Contrast-enhanced apical four-chamber view during diastole showing focal increase in myocardial thickness at the apex (*arrows*) giving a "spade" like appearance to the LV cavity.

- Inject saline flush SLOWLY; otherwise this will cause apical contrast attenuation.
- Follow with a 1 mL Slow flush.
- Repeat as needed. Increase or decrease injection rate based on image quality.

## PREPARING OPTISON™ (GE HEALTHCARE) CONTRAST

- Draw up 3 mL of Optison™ with a vented spike and dilute in 5 mL of saline
- Suspend the solution until milky by rolling between the palms of your hands
- Lower MI to 0.3 to 0.4
- Inject 1 to 2 mL of Optison™ solution followed by a **SLOW** saline flush
- Change gain settings to optimize endocardial border detection
- Repeat as needed. Increase or decrease injection rate based on image quality

## PITFALLS

### High Mechanical Index:
- This disrupts and destroys the contrast microbubbles.
- This is seen as a dark swirling artifact especially close to where the ultrasound beam is focused.
- To fix → decrease MI and re-inject contrast slowly.

### Attenuation:
- Caused by injecting contrast too fast or pushing too much.
- This is seen as a bright "pool" of contrast in the apex that casts a shadow over the rest of the heart.

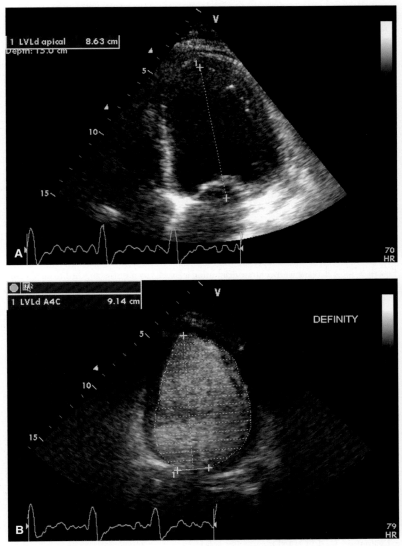

**Figure 3-3.** The difference in accuracy in measuring LV volume and long-axis dimensions between **(A)** unenhanced end-diastolic apical four-chamber and **(B)** contrast-enhanced end-diastolic apical four-chamber view.

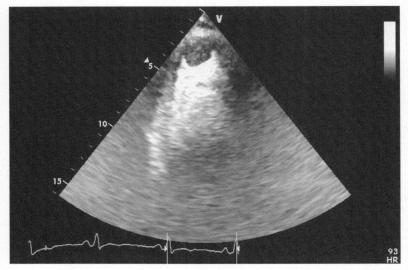

**Figure 3-4.** A2C view with contrast delineating a "black" ovoid mass attached to an akinetic LV apex consistent with thrombus.

- To fix → either wait for some of the contrast to transit through the heart or move the focus point to the apex and turn the MI up to destroy some of the bubbles. Then turn the MI back down and return the focus point back to the base of the heart (Fig. 3-5).

### LV Underfilled with Contrast:
- Especially seen affecting the apex or in patients with dilated LV (Fig. 3-6).
- This is seen as "swirling" of contrast as it mixes with unopacified blood in the LV.
- To fix → Inject more contrast then flush with a faster flush. This will help push the contrast to the apex.

## AGITATED BACTERIOSTATIC SALINE CONTRAST

### Reasons to Perform an Agitated Saline Contrast:
- Patients who have unexplained right heart enlargement
- Patients with suspected TIA or CVA (<55 years of age)
- Evaluation for PFO/ASD
- Atrial septal aneurysm
- Enhance TR jet for PA systolic pressure measurement (not as accurate as using commercially available contrasts because of spectral broadening)

### Contraindications:
- Known VSD
- Pregnancy

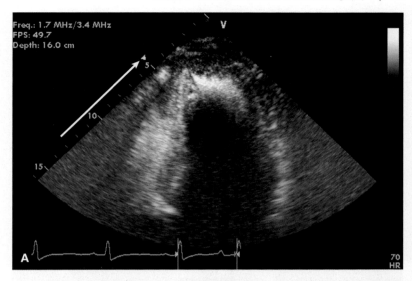

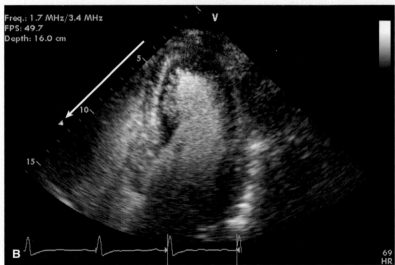

Figure 3-5. **A:** Pooling of the contrast in the LV apex causing attenuation of the basal to mid LV cavity in this apical four-chamber view. The focus (▷) is transiently shifted to the apex to "destroy" excess bubbles and allow the proximal chamber to be visualized. The focus can then be re-adjusted back to the normal position at the base of the heart **(B)**.

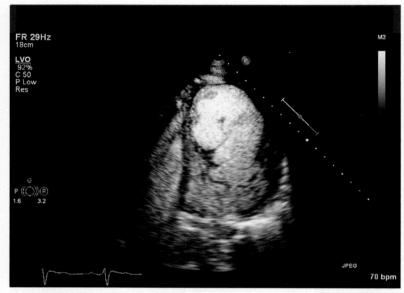

**Figure 3-6.** Swirling unenhanced blood is seen in a dilated LV secondary to inadequate amount of contrast injected.

## PREPARING AGITATED BACTERIOSTATIC SALINE CONTRAST

If patients have both contrast and agitated saline contrast ordered, the saline contrast should be given for evaluation of shunt before contrast is used!

- Draw 8 mL bacteriostatic saline into a 10 mL syringe, connect to a three-way stop-cock and connect an empty 10 mL syringe to the other port.
- Leave 1 mL of air in the saline syringe, but ensure that there is no air in the IV line or stop-cock.
- Agitate the solution (with stop-cock in closed position to patient) by rapidly transferring the volume of one syringe to the other, back and forth several times until the solution is foamy.
- Inject the agitated saline.
- Repeat injection with patient performing Valsalva maneuver.
- Capture 8 to 10 beat loops of both normal and Valsalva injections (long capture is important to evaluate for extra-cardiac shunts).

## INJECTION OF AGITATED SALINE

- Typically performed for detection of cardiac shunts.
- Saline "bubbles" are in general too large to pass through the pulmonary circulation and opacify the left heart, unless a right-to-left shunt bypassing the pulmonary capillary bed is present.
- Shunts are defined as intra-cardiac at the level of the atria (PFO, ASD) or extra-cardiac (pulmonary or hepatic arterial-venous malformations).

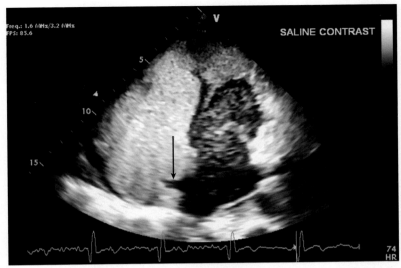

**Figure 3-7.** Apical four chamber with injected saline bubble study showing "negative contrast" (*arrow*) in RA secondary to L→R shunt.

- Left-to-right shunts may be seen as **"negative"** contrast in the RA where non-opacified blood from the LA is outlined by the injected agitated saline in the RA (Fig. 3-7).
- If persistent left superior vena cava (PLSVC) is suspected then the bubble study should be performed from an IV placed in the left arm and opacification should be observed from a PLAX view. The coronary sinus will opacify before the RV if PLSVC is present (Fig. 3-8).

---

- **Key Point:** *The following features after saline injection suggest (a) intra-cardiac shunt–quick, dense opacification of LV (<3 to 4 beats) – opacification is intensified or occurs only with Valsalva (PFO), if shunt is significant RV enlargement may be present (ASD); (b) extra-cardiac shunt–delayed opacification (>5 to 6 beats) – opacification slowly builds in intensity in the LV with each successive beat as the bubbles slowly circulate to the LV, site of bubble entry into LA is pulmonary veins.*

---

- **Key Point:** *"Pseudocontrast" (faint, diffuse bubbles), may be seen transiently (1 to 2 beats) in the LA and LV, unrelated to injection of agitated saline, secondary to the release of "stagnant" blood in the pulmonary veins after Valsalva causing spontaneous echo contrast. This can be confirmed by repeating Valsalva without agitated saline injection to reproduce the "pseudocontrast" effect. In contrast false negative agitated saline studies may be related to the inability to transiently increase RA pressure above LA pressure (e.g., inadequate Valsalva, severe LV diastolic dysfunction) or antecubital vein injection of agitated saline being directed away from the inter-atrial septum especially in the presence of a prominent eustachian valve. In this latter case femoral injection of agitated saline may be required to rule out the presence of an inter-atrial shunt.*

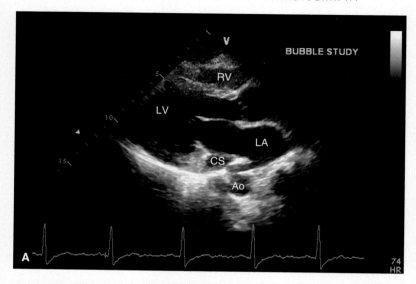

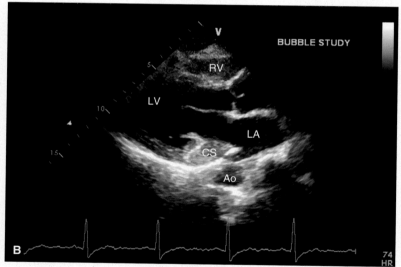

Figure 3-8. Patient with persistent left SVC with bubble study performed from IV in left arm. A: PLAX prior to injection showing a dilated coronary sinus. B: Early after injection of agitated saline, PLAX showing opacification of the CS before the RV. C: Later after injection of agitated saline, PLAX showing opacification of both CS and RV.

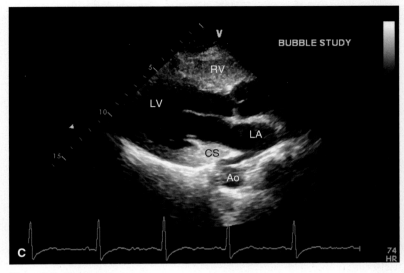

**Figure 3.8.** (*Continued*)

# 4

# Quantification of Left Ventricular Systolic and Diastolic Function

Christopher L. Holley

HIGH-YIELD FINDINGS

- *Normal LV size:* PLAX diameter <5.3 cm ♀, 5.9 cm ♂; apical four-chamber end diastolic volume indexed to BSA ≤75 mL/m$^2$
- *Normal LV systolic function:* Ejection fraction ≥55%
- *Normal LV mass indexed to BSA:* <89 mL/m$^2$ ♀, <103 mL/m$^2$ ♂
- *Normal LA size indexed to BSA:* <22 +/− 6 mL/m$^2$
- *Normal diastolic function* is quickly assessed by TDI of the mitral annulus; e′ lateral ≥10 cm/s or medial ≥8 cm/s

KEY VIEWS

- *Parasternal long axis:* 2D (linear) measurements of LV, LA, and aortic root
- *Parasternal short axis:* Assessment of LV mass
- *Apical four chamber:* Tracings for LV and LA volumes; Doppler assessment of mitral inflow and annular velocities

## INTRODUCTION

Accurate quantitative assessment of the left ventricle (LV) is an essential aspect of echocardiography. At the time of interpretation, indexed measurements (to BSA or height) should be used in reports, as "normal" measurements vary significantly by gender and body size.

### Tips for Optimizing Image Quality:

- Adjust image acquisition settings as detailed in Chapter 1. Optimizing patient positioning and acquiring images at held end-expiration may also improve image quality.
- Use contrast (see Chapter 3) when appropriate to visualize the endocardium (i.e., unable to assess ≥2 myocardial segments).

### Tips for Interpreting Studies:

- *Qualitative* size and function estimates should be avoided except as a "reality check" for measured values.
- Use *multiple views* for assessment.

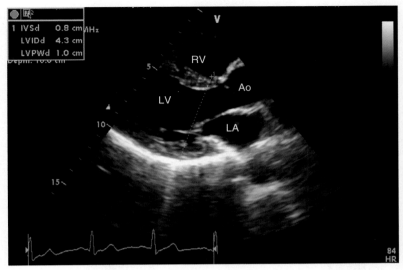

**Figure 4-1.** Parasternal long-axis view with linear left ventricular measurements performed at the level of the mitral valve leaflet tips.

- Beware of *off-axis* views as they may distort the comparative size of chambers and not allow use of standardized normal ranges.

## LV DIMENSIONS

- Parasternal long axis (PLAX)
  - At a minimum, make simple linear measurements and compare to (non-indexed) upper limits of normal (Fig. 4-1 and Table 4-1)
    - LVID ("minor axis," LVIDd and LVIDs, measured at MV leaflet tips in end-diastole and end-systole respectively)
    - Septal and inferolateral wall thicknesses (measured at MV leaflet tips in end-diastole)

| TABLE 4-1 | Linear Dimensions | | | | |
|---|---|---|---|---|---|
| | LVIDd (cm) | SWT or PWT (cm) | RWT | Aorta (cm) | LA (cm) |
| **Upper normal** | 5.3 ♀, 5.9 ♂ | 1 | 0.42 | 4[a] | 4 |
| **Severely abnormal** | ≥6.3 | ≥1.7 | ≥0.53 | § | ≥5.2 |

[a]Indicates wide variance with age and BSA. (Adapted from Lang RM, Bierig M, Devereux RB, et al. Recommendations for chamber quantification: a report from the American Society of Echocardiography's Guidelines and Standards Committee and the Chamber Quantification Writing Group, developed in conjunction with the European Association of Echocardiography, a branch of the European Society of Cardiology. *J Am Soc Echocardiogr.* 2005;18:1440–1463). § See Figure 4-2.

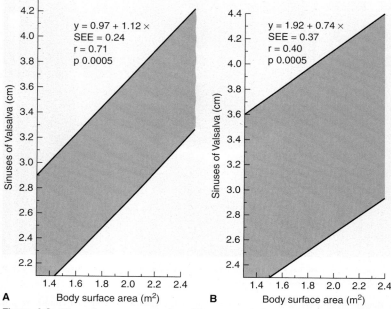

**Figure 4-2.** Ninety-five percent normal confidence intervals for aortic root dimension at the sinuses of Valsalva indexed to body surface area for adults <40 years of age **(A)** and those ≥40 years **(B)**. (Reprinted from Roman MJ, Devereux RB, Kramer-Fox R, et al. Two-dimensional echocardiographic aortic root dimensions in normal children and adults. *Am J Cardiol.* 1989;64:507–512, with permission from Elsevier.)

- ○ Aortic (Ao) root diameter, at the sinuses, sinotubular junction and proximal ascending aorta (see Chapters 9 and 10) (Fig. 4-2)
- ○ LA size is more accurately measured as a volume in the A4C rather than linear dimensions in the PLAX view
- M-mode measurements may be used although beware of errors related to beam angle (Fig. 4-3)
- Apical views (A4C and A2C)
  - The minimum assessment should include LA volume assessment and measurement of LV volume in systole and diastole for LV ejection fraction (Table 4-2)
    - ○ The LA is measured at end-systole tracing from the MV annulus and excluding the pulmonary veins and LA appendage.
    - ○ The LV volume tracing should exclude the papillary muscles and trabeculations. Ensure that a *non-foreshortened* view is used (apex should move inward rather than toward the annulus).
    - ○ The LV long-axis length at end-diastole is also used in the calculation of LV mass and is another method to ensure that images are not foreshortened.

---

- **Key Point:** *Use of contrast does not increase accuracy of chamber measurements if the apical images are foreshortened. Optimize probe and patient positioning before injection of contrast and reduction of machine mechanical index.*

---

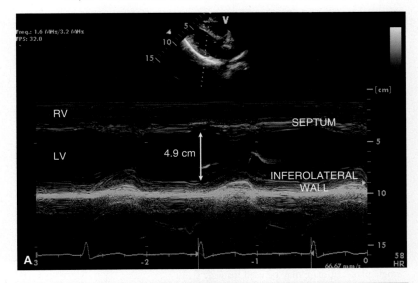

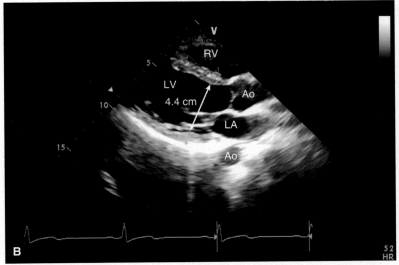

Figure 4-3. (A) M-mode oblique to long axis of the LV in the PLAX view leading to overestimation of the LV end-diastolic internal diameter compared to 2D measurement (B) in same patient.

| TABLE 4-2 | Volumes and Mass | | | |
|---|---|---|---|---|
| | LA volume indexed to BSA (mL/m²) | LV diastolic volume indexed to BSA (mL/m²) | LV systolic volume indexed to BSA (mL/m²) | LV mass by 2D method indexed to BSA (g/m²) |
| **Upper normal** | 29 | 75 | 30 | 88 |
| **Severely abnormal** | ≥40 | ≥97 | ≥43 | ≥131 |

Adapted from Lang RM, Bierig M, Devereux RB, et al. Recommendations for chamber quantification: a report from the American Society of Echocardiography's Guidelines and Standards Committee and the Chamber Quantification Writing Group, developed in conjunction with the European Association of Echocardiography, a branch of the European Society of Cardiology. *J Am Soc Echocardiogr.* 2005;18:1440–1463.

## LV SYSTOLIC FUNCTION

- The preferred method is the modified Simpson's biplane estimate (summation of elliptical discs along LV long axis; formula not shown but available in standard analysis packages) (Table 4-3). If there are no regional wall motion abnormalities a single plane estimate may be used instead.
  - Biplane method: Use A4C and A2C views to trace LV volumes for end-systole and end-diastole
  - Single plane method: Use A4C or A2C view to trace LV volumes for end-systole and end-diastole (Fig. 4-4)
  - EF = (EDV − ESV)/EDV
- LVEF is not only influenced by intrinsic myocardial function *but also LV geometry*. For example, patients with concentric LVH may have a normal or even increased LVEF but significant intrinsic myocardial dysfunction. This is because LVEF relies on inward endocardial displacement that is independently affected by RWT. LV strain measurements can uncover intrinsic myocardial dysfunction *independent of LV geometry*. Systolic strain describes how the myocardium deforms by comparing the original myocardial length ($L_o$) at end-diastole to its final length ($L_f$) at end-systole ($L_f − L_o/L_o$). 2D-LV strain tracks the intrinsic inhomogeneities or "speckles" in the myocardium to measure these changes. From the three apical views a global or mean peak systolic strain can be calculated as an indicator of global LV systolic function (Fig. 4-4C). The influence of artifact on strain measurements has limited its clinical application.

## LV MASS

- 2D methods are preferred (Fig. 4-5A and B)
  - Area-length (use SAX epicardial/endocardial areas to determine myocardial thickness, plus LV long axis from A4C) assumes the LV shape is a prolate ellipse

| TABLE 4-3 | LV Functional Assessment | |
|---|---|---|
| | LVEF (%) | 2D-Peak global longitudinal strain (mean,%) |
| **Normal** | ≥55% | ≤−18.6%[a] |

[a]Negative sign denotes shortening; that is, more negative numbers = increased shortening.

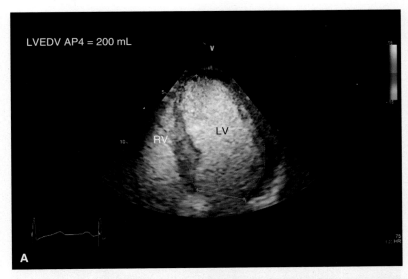

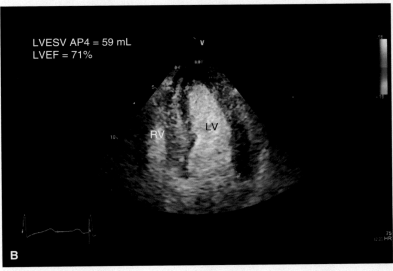

Figure 4-4. Quantifying left ventricular systolic function in a patient with left ventricular hypertrophy by calculating LVEF using the single plane modified Simpson's method (**A, B**) and global 2D longitudinal peak strain (GLPS) (**C**). Note despite normal LVEF (71%) there is a marked reduction in GLPS (−14%).(*continued*)

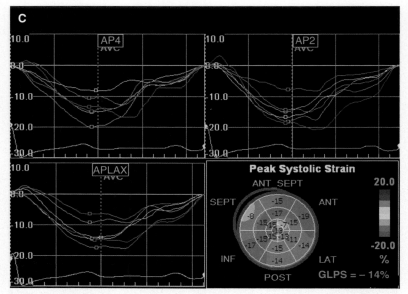

Figure 4-4. (*Continued*)

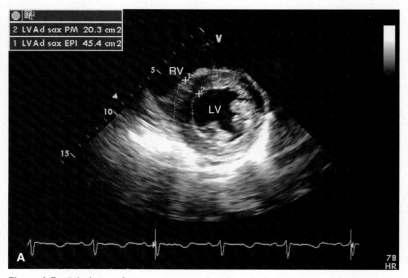

Figure 4-5. Calculation of LV mass using area-length method. **(A)** Parasternal short axis at the mid-LV level with tracing of endocardium (excluding papillary muscles) and epicardium.

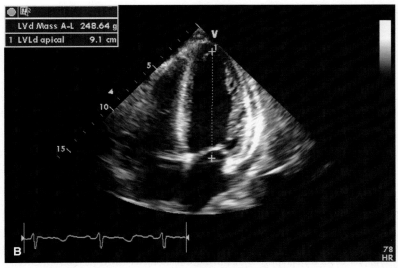

**Figure 4-5.** (*Continued*) **(B)** Apical four-chamber with LV long-axis measurement at end-diastole from mitral annulus to LV apex.

- Truncated ellipsoid method (need the above, *plus* A4C MV annular width) used when significant distortion to LV shape is present.
- Calculations automated on most machines
- Linear method: Use left ventricular internal diameter at end-diastole (LVIDd), septal wall thickness (SWT), inferolateral wall thickness (ILWT) from PLAX view
  - LV mass = $0.8 \times (1.04 \, [(LVIDd + ILWT + SWT)^3 - (LVID)^3]) + 0.6$ g
  - Characterization of hypertrophy is based on relative wall thickness (RWT) from PLAX in conjunction with calculated LV mass (indexed to body surface area) (Table 4-4). RWT indexes wall thickness to the long-axis dimension of the ventricle.
  - RWT = $2 \times$ ILWT/LVIDd

| TABLE 4-4 | Relationships Between LV Mass and RWT | |
| --- | --- | --- |
| | **LVMI ≤95 ♀, 115 ♂** | **LVMI >95 ♀, 115 ♂** |
| **RWT ≤0.42** | Normal | Eccentric hypertrophy |
| **RWT >0.42** | Concentric remodeling | Concentric hypertrophy |

LVMI, LV mass indexed to BSA (g/m$^2$).

Adapted from Lang RM, Bierig M, Devereux RB, et al. Recommendations for chamber quantification: a report from the American Society of Echocardiography's Guidelines and Standards Committee and the Chamber Quantification Writing Group, developed in conjunction with the European Association of Echocardiography, a branch of the European Society of Cardiology. *J Am Soc Echocardiogr.* 2005;18:1440–1463.

| TABLE 4-5 | Quantitative Limits for Indices Used to Categorize Stages of Diastolic Dysfunction | | | |
|---|---|---|---|---|
| **Classification** | | Grade 1 | Grade 2 | Grades 3/4 |
| | **Normal** | **Impaired** | **Pseudonormal** | **Restrictive** |
| E/A | ≥0.8 | <0.8 | 0.8–1.5 | >2 |
| DT (ms) | <200 | >200 | 160–200 | ≤160 |
| e′ lateral (cm/s) | ≥10 | ≥10 | <10 | <10 |
| e′ septal (cm/s) | ≥8 | ≥8 | <8 | <8 |
| E/e′ (septal) | ≤8 | ≤8 | 9–14 | ≥15 |
| E/e′ (lateral) | ≤8 | ≤8 | 9–14 | ≥12 |
| E/e′ (average) | ≤8 | ≤8 | 9–14 | ≥13 |

Adapted from Nagueh SF, Appleton CP, Gillebert TC, et al. Recommendations for the evaluation of left ventricular diastolic function by echocardiography. *J Am Soc Echocardiogr.* 2009;22:107–133.

## DIASTOLIC ASSESSMENT

See Table 4-5 and Figure 4-6.

- Doppler echocardiography, unlike invasive manometer based methods, indirectly measures LV diastolic function through changes that occur in the pressure gradients between the LA and LV
- Mitral inflow pulsed-wave (PW) Doppler: E and A waves
  - A4C view, PW Doppler at MV leaflet tips
  - Key parameters:
    ○ E = peak early mitral inflow velocity
    ○ A = peak late mitral inflow velocity
    ○ DT = deceleration time (time from peak E velocity to baseline)
    ○ IVRT = isovolumic relaxation time (time between aortic valve closure and mitral valve opening)
  - Normally filling occurs predominantly early in diastole because of rapid LV relaxation that "sucks" blood from the LA; that is, E > A
  - Impairment of myocardial relaxation leads to a reliance on filling during late diastole; that is, E < A
  - In more severe stages of diastolic dysfunction as LA pressure rises in response to ineffective filling, this ratio may "normalize". LA blood is "pushed" into the LV; that is, E > A (pseudonormal) or E >> A (restrictive)
  - Aging itself leads to gradual diastolic impairment, such that E = A by around age 65 (E/A = 1), with E < A by age 70
  - The strain phase of Valsalva may be used to unmask underlying impaired myocardial relaxation in patients with a "pseudonormal pattern" by transiently reducing LA filling pressure. Similarly this may be seen in "reversible" restrictive filling patterns. The use of this technique has been limited by the variability in patient effort to effect a reduction in LA pressure.
  - IVRT and DT lengthen with impaired myocardial relaxation as the rate of LV pressure decline is reduced in early diastole; therefore, reducing the transmitral filling gradient (loss of "suction"). In more severe diastolic dysfunction, IVRT and DT will shorten, secondary to a marked rise in LA driving pressure and reduced LV compliance (increase in "pushing").

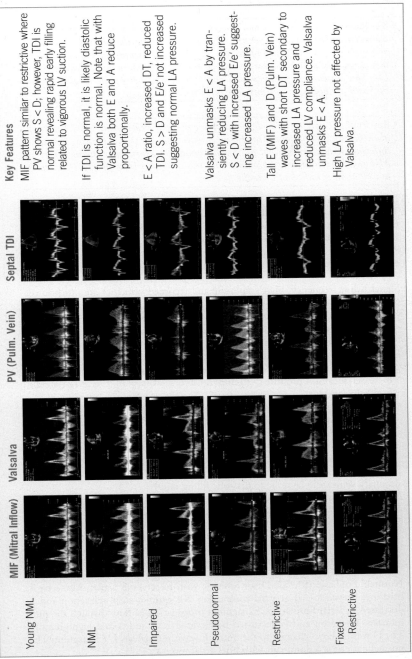

**Key Features**

|  | MIF (Mitral Inflow) | Valsalva | PV (Pulm. Vein) | Septal TDI | Key Features |
|---|---|---|---|---|---|
| Young NML | | | | | MIF pattern similar to restrictive where PV shows S < D; however, TDI is normal revealing rapid early filling related to vigorous LV suction. |
| NML | | | | | If TDI is normal, it is likely diastolic function is normal. Note that with Valsalva both E and A reduce proportionally. |
| Impaired | | | | | E < A ratio, increased DT, reduced TDI. S > D and E/e' not increased suggesting normal LA pressure. |
| Pseudonormal | | | | | Valsalva unmasks E < A by transiently reducing LA pressure. S < D with increased E/e' suggesting increased LA pressure. |
| Restrictive | | | | | Tall E (MIF) and D (Pulm. Vein) waves with short DT secondary to increased LA pressure and reduced LV compliance. Valsalva unmasks E < A. |
| Fixed Restrictive | | | | | High LA pressure not affected by Valsalva. |

**Figure 4-6.** Use of diastolic function indices to categorize stage of diastolic dysfunction.

51

> • **Key Point:** *Vigorous LV "suction" suggests normal diastolic function with active LV relaxation and a compliant ventricle drawing blood from the LA under low filling pressures. The need to "push" blood into the LV suggests significant diastolic dysfunction as now filling pressures are elevated in order to move blood into a non-compliant LV. This is seen with pseudonormal and restrictive Doppler patterns and portends increased morbidity for patients with heart failure.*

> • **Key Point:** *It may be difficult to determine diastolic function using MIF patterns alone because—(a) fusion of the E and A waves may not allow analysis, (b) cannot differentiate between normal or "pseudonormal" or restrictive patterns. Therefore MIF should be used in combination with tissue Doppler imaging (TDI) especially, as well as other indices of Diastolic function.*

- TDI of the mitral annulus
  - **The most sensitive and reliable echocardiographic index of diastolic function, as long as there are no localized influences affecting annular motion. Rely on this parameter more than any other.**
  - A4C view, PW Doppler sample volume on septal or lateral MV annulus
  - $e'$ = tissue Doppler velocity of mitral annulus; normal septal $\geq 8$ cm/s, lateral $\geq 10$ cm/s
  - Signal is low frequency, high amplitude and recorded velocities are much lower than blood flow velocities
    - Lateral annulus velocity is usually greater than septal annulus (exceptions include any regional influences on annular motion such as constrictive pericarditis)
    - Less affected by preload than MIF
  - Ratio of $E/e'$ correlates with LA pressure
    - Normal LA pressure: $E/e' \leq 8$ (septal, lateral, or average of both)
    - Increased mean LA pressure (>20 mmHg): $E/e' \geq 15$ (septal), $E/e' \geq 12$ (lateral), $E/e' \geq 13$ (average)
    - $E/e'$ = 9–14 are indeterminate values but may be associated with elevated LA pressure if any of the following additional features of elevated filling pressures are present: LA volume $\geq 34$ mL/m$^2$, pulmonary artery systolic pressure >35 mmHg (in patients without primary pulmonary disease), change in E/A ratio with Valsalva $\geq 0.5$, pulmonary S < D wave peak velocities, pulmonary atrial reversal duration (Ar) exceeds mitral A duration $\geq 30$ ms (see below)
- Pulmonary veins: S/D (systolic to diastolic filling ratio)
  - A4C view, PW Doppler at atrial "back wall" (right superior pulmonary vein)

> • **Key Point:** *The right superior pulmonary vein is located near the inter-atrial septum and is best aligned for parallel Doppler interrogation. Slight anterior angulation of the probe (almost to an Apical five-chamber) offers best visualization of the vein. This is vital to obtain a good quality Doppler profile.*

- Normal: Triphasic (S1, S2, D) or biphasic with fusion of S waves. Also seen is brief atrial reversal (Ar) at atrial contraction. S1 signifies atrial relaxation and is decreased in atrial fibrillation, S2 signifies propagation of flow through the pulmonary circulation and is decreased by elevated LAP and mitral regurgitation. The D wave follows changes to the mitral E wave and reflects LV relaxation. The normal pattern is S dominant with brief atrial reversal.

- Abnormal filling pressures: As mean LA pressure rises, filling during ventricular systole diminishes and the atrium fills primarily during early ventricular diastole (S < D). With reduced LV compliance there is an increase in LVEDP and Ar duration (≥30 ms longer than mitral A wave duration) and amplitude (>35 cm/s) (i.e., blood refluxes back into pulmonary veins with atrial contraction with increasing LV filling pressures).

---

- **Key Point:** *Despite Doppler echocardiography being the main modality for evaluating diastolic function, always place these measurements in the context of the 2D images; for example, diastolic function is unlikely to be normal if there is significant LVH, cardiomyopathy and LA enlargement. Use 2D imaging to corroborate Doppler findings of increased LA pressure and also to identify reasons why Doppler indices may be discrepant and not reflective of LV diastolic function, such as significant mitral annular calcification or adherent pericardium limiting mitral annular motion.*

---

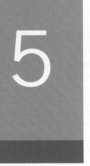

# 5 Right Ventricular Function and Pulmonary Hemodynamics

Suzanne V. Arnold

## HIGH-YIELD FINDINGS

- *Right ventricular size* should be << left ventricular (LV) size
- *RV dysfunction*—decreased tricuspid valve (TV) annular motion, RV outflow duration << TR duration
- *RV pressure* overload—systolic interventricular septal flattening, high-velocity tricuspid regurgitant (TR) jet, short right ventricular outflow tract (RVOT) acceleration time, RVOT outflow notching
- *RV volume* overload—diastolic interventricular septal flattening, severe pulmonic regurgitation (PR)
- *Right atrial (RA) pressure* increase—dilated inferior vena cava (IVC), interatrial septal bowing to left

## KEY VIEWS

- *Parasternal long axis and RV inflow*—initial screening of RA/RV size and TR jet
- *Parasternal short axis*—assessment of interventricular septal flattening, TR jet, RVOT outflow pattern, PR jet
- *Apical four chamber*—best view for RA/RV size, qualitative RV function, tricuspid valve (TV), annular motion, TR jet, interatrial septum
- *Subcostal*—assessment of RVH and IVC

## ANATOMY AND PHYSIOLOGY OF THE RIGHT VENTRICLE

- The RV is fundamentally different from the LV in both structure and function such that methods typically used to assess the LV do **not** work for the RV.
- The RV is a **thin-walled pyramidal structure** that "wraps around" the LV. The RV is divided into two sections: Inflow (TV, papillary muscles, chordae tendinae, myocardium) and outflow (conus or infundibulum and pulmonic valve [PV]). Additional structures unique to the RV: Crista supraventricularis, prominent trabeculations, moderator band.
- In contrast to the LV, the RV is **highly compliant and energetically-efficient; designed to pump blood into the low-resistance, high-capacitance pulmonary circulation**. The RV is less capable of maintaining stroke volume in the setting of acute increases in afterload.

- The RV contracts by three separate mechanisms: Inward movement of the free wall to the interventricular septum (i.e., "bellows" motion: This allows for a large volume shift with little transverse motion), contraction of longitudinal fibers, and traction on the free wall due to LV contraction. This method of contraction is fundamentally different than that of the LV. The main driving force of the LV comes from a layer of circumferential constrictor fibers that act to reduce ventricular diameter. The RV lacks these fibers and thus must rely more heavily on longitudinal shortening than does the LV. In addition, although the RV does undergo torsion, this does not contribute substantially to RV contraction.
- The **RV and LV are interdependent,** with common encircling muscle fibers, a shared interventricular septum, and the pericardium. It is estimated that ~65% of RV pressure and volume outflow are generated by the LV.

## RV SIZE AND FUNCTION

### 2D Assessment

- Important to assess in patients with pulmonary embolism, pulmonary hypertension, RV infarction, LV assist devices, congenital heart disease.
- The RV is a complex 3D shape and unlike the LV is difficult to model with a single 2D echocardiographic view. Therefore **multiple** views should be assessed before determining that RV enlargement is present.
- *Qualitative:* A standard apical four-chamber (A4C) view is best to assess RV size as compared to LV.
  - Mildly enlarged: RV is enlarged but <LV
  - Moderately enlarged: RV ≈ LV
  - Severely enlarged: RV > LV. Apex of heart comprised of RV
- *Quantitative:*
  - PLAX RVOT proximal diameter >3.3 cm
  - PSAX RVOT distal diameter >2.7 cm
  - Apical four-chamber RV basal diameter in diastole >4.2 cm
- As RV enlarges, it assumes more of a spherical shape and can impair LV output (Fig. 5-1).

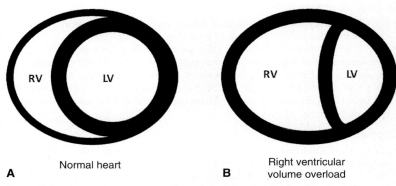

**A** Normal heart  **B** Right ventricular volume overload

Figure 5-1. Changes in normal LV and RV shape **(A)** with RV volume overload **(B)**.

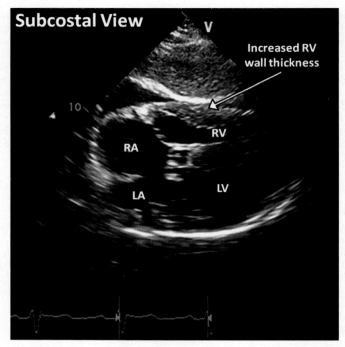

**Figure 5-2.** A subcostal image showing clear delineation of the borders of the hypertrophied RV wall. For accurate measurement, a zoomed 2D view or M-mode should be acquired.

---

- **Key Point:** *It is critical that qualitative assessment of RV size be made in standard transducer locations. If the transducer is placed too medially in the apical four-chamber view, the RV will always appear larger.*

---

### M-mode Assessment

- RV wall thickness measured at peak of R wave on electrocardiogram at level of TV chordae in subcostal view (normal ≤5 mm) (Fig. 5-2).
- As RV systolic function primarily relies on longitudinal myocardial shortening, measurement of tricuspid annular plane systolic excursion (**TAPSE**) can be used. In the apical four-chamber view, an M-mode cursor is oriented to the junction of the TV plane with the RV free wall. TAPSE is the difference in the displacement of the RV base during diastole and systole. **Abnormal excursion <1.7 cm** (low sensitivity but high specificity) (Fig. 5-3).

### Doppler Assessment

- RV function can be assessed by the myocardial performance index (**MPI**) or **Tei index,** which is the ratio of isovolumic time to ventricular ejection time. It is a measure of **both systolic and diastolic function**. For this measurement the TR jet duration (CW Doppler) and RVOT jet duration (PW Doppler) are

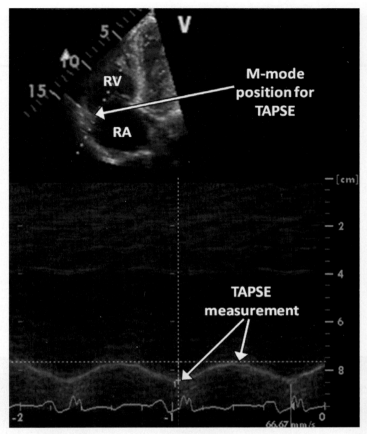

**Figure 5-3.** Using M-mode positioned from the RV apex through the RV free wall and tricuspid annulus intersection to measure TAPSE.

recorded. Since TR occurs from a high to low pressure chamber (i.e., RV → RA), flow is **holosystolic**—including isovolumic contraction and relaxation times. Thus, to determine isovolumic time, subtract ejection time from TR duration (Fig. 5-4).

- MPI = (isovolumic contraction time [IVCT] + isovolumic relaxation time [IVRT])/ejection time; IVCT + IVRT = TR time – RVOT ejection time.
  - **MPI = (TR time – RVOT ejection time)/RVOT ejection time**
  - **Normal <0.4.** Value increases with systolic and diastolic RV dysfunction.

Tissue Doppler imaging can also be used for quantitative assessment of RV systolic function. **Systolic tissue Doppler signal of the lateral TV annulus (Sa) <10 cm/s suggests RV dysfunction** (Fig. 5-5).

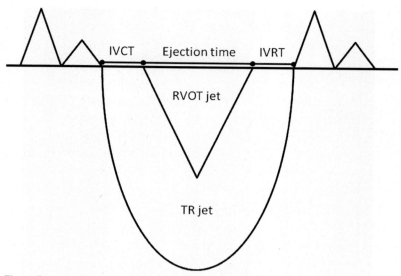

**Figure 5-4.** A cartoon superimposing RVOT and TR Doppler jets to demonstrate the intervals measured for calculation of RV MPI.

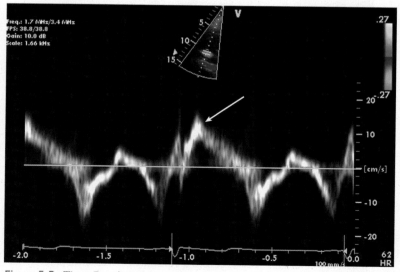

**Figure 5-5.** Tissue Doppler imaging of the lateral tricuspid annulus demonstrating normal systolic peak velocity ~11.5 cm/s (*arrow*).

## RV PATHOLOGY

### RV Volume Overload

- Typically seen as a result of **L → R shunt** (atrial septal defect [ASD], anomalous pulmonary venous return, arteriovenous malformation) or severe pulmonary insufficiency (Fig. 5-6).

> - **Key Point:** *In contrast to an ASD, patients with a ventricular septal defect (VSD), initially develop LV volume overload (**not the RV**) as the blood is moved into the pulmonary circulation and thus the RV does not "see" the extra volume.*

- Classic findings are a dilated RV with **diastolic interventricular septal flattening** (Fig. 5-6). ASD flow is best seen in the subcostal view by reducing the Nyquist limit and when Doppler interrogation is parallel to flow. This is typically low velocity (~2 m/s) with the Doppler envelope showing a broad peak in late systole and early diastole and a small terminal peak with atrial contraction. With substantial L→R shunt, there will be increased flows across all valves distal to the shunt (i.e., increased TV and PV flows).
- Signs of concomitant **increased right heart pressure** may also be seen.

### RV Pressure Overload

- Results from **high pulmonary artery pressures, pulmonary stenosis, or when the RV is the systemic ventricle in congenital heart disease**. Acute increases in PA pressures, as seen in acute pulmonary embolism, can cause RV failure, as the RV cannot adapt quickly to changes in afterload. With chronically elevated PA pressures, the RV hypertrophies, spherically remodels and can maintain systolic function at higher pressures than seen in the acute setting.

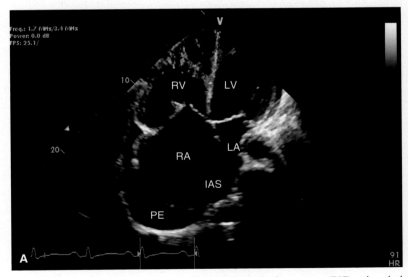

**Figure 5-6.** Patient with arteriovenous malformation(right lumbar artery to IVC) and marked RV volume overload. **(A)** Apical four chamber with massive RA and RV dilatation and bowing of interatrial septum to the LA. Small, medium posterior pericardial effusion (PE) seen. (*continued*)

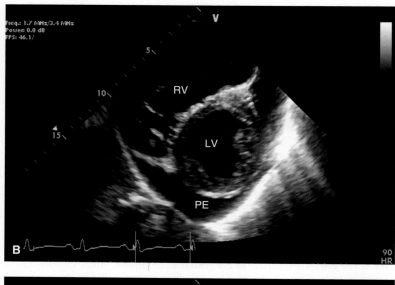

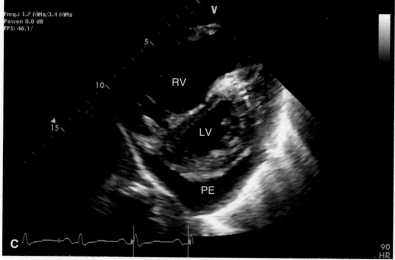

Figure 5-6. (*Continued*) (**B**) Parasternal short-axis view in systole with paradoxical interventricular septal motion. (**C**) Parasternal short-axis view in diastole with diastolic septal flattening.

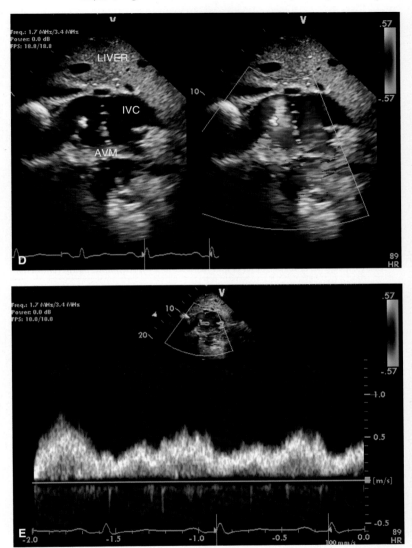

**Figure 5-6.** (*Continued*) **(D)** Side-by-side subcostal view of the dilated IVC with color Doppler showing communication and a larger area of flow from the posterior lumbar artery. **(E)** Spectral Doppler of the shunt shows a continuous dense envelope.

- RV pressures can be estimated using the TR jet and the RV outflow pattern. In the absence of a gradient across the pulmonary valve (i.e., pulmonary stenosis), **RV pressure estimates PA pressure**.
- Qualitative signs of high PA pressures: **Dilated pulmonary arteries** (>3 cm in the parasternal short axis at the level of the AoV is markedly abnormal), **RV hypertrophy** (>5 mm at level of TV chordae in subcostal view at end-diastole is abnormal), **systolic interventricular septum flattening** (i.e., "D-shaped" LV; best seen in parasternal short axis at level of papillary muscles indicates marked increase in RV pressure to near systemic levels), **high velocity TR jet, short RVOT acceleration time** (<90 ms)**, shortened RVOT TVI, mid-systolic closure of pulmonic valve flow.**

---

- **Key Point:** *"60:60 sign"—In the setting of an acute pulmonary embolism, the RVOT acceleration time may be shortened (<60 ms), secondary to local fluid hemodynamic changes and does not accurately reflect mean PA pressure. This phenomenon is confirmed by a low velocity TR jet, reflecting only a modest increase in peak PA systolic pressure (<60 mmHg gradient).*

---

- **Key Point:** *McConnell's sign—In addition to changes in pulmonary hemodynamics, acute pulmonary embolism can produce regional RV wall motion abnormalities, with severe hypokinesis of the RV basal to mid free wall and hyperdynamic apical contraction.*

---

## RV Infarction

- If the ECG is concerning for acute inferior myocardial infarction (MI), particularly if **ST segment elevations in lead III > lead II or are seen in right sided precordial leads,** obtain a careful assessment of RV function by echocardiography.
- Typical findings would be **hypokinesis/akinesis of the inferior LV wall in addition to the RV.** Quantitative evidence of RV dysfunction—high RV MPI, low TAPSE—without chronic changes (no RV hypertrophy, normal to mildly elevated PA pressures).
- Clinically, these patients are **preload-dependent.** Volume depletion and nitroglycerin can precipitate profound hypotension.

### Arrhythmogenic Right Ventricular Dysplasia

Arrhythmogenic right ventricular dysplasia (ARVD) is a rare congenital disorder involving focal or diffuse replacement of RV myocardium with adipose tissue. This clinically manifests as syncope or sudden cardiac death resulting from ventricular tachycardia originating from these abnormal areas of infiltration. Echocardiographic findings are **RV enlargement, free wall thinning, focal aneurysms, and systolic dysfunction.** Aneurysms are most frequently seen in the RV basal inferior, apical, and anterior outflow walls. The LV is normal in ARVD, in contrast to the case of RV infarction. Absence of the above findings does not exclude this diagnosis.


## PULMONARY HEMODYNAMICS

### Estimating PA Pressure

- **PA systolic and diastolic pressure can be estimated using the modified Bernoulli equation,** which calculates the pressure difference between two chambers of the heart using the velocity of a jet between them. $\Delta P$ (measured in mmHg) = 4 × $V^2$ (measured in m/s) (see Chapter 1).

- To estimate RV systolic pressure (which estimates PA systolic pressure [PASP] in the absence of a gradient across the RVOT/PV), try to obtain the TR jet in multiple views: Parasternal long-axis/RV inflow, parasternal short axis at level of AoV, apical four-chamber, and subcostal views. Use the highest velocity TR jet where the Doppler envelope is *complete, measuring the modal peak velocity (darkest part of jet).*
  - $\Delta P = 4 \times V^2$
  - RV systolic pressure – RA pressure = $4 \times$ (peak velocity of TR jet)$^2$
  - **PASP $\approx 4 \times$ (peak velocity of TR jet)$^2$ + mean RA pressure**
  - **Normal PASP <35 mmHg**

  ---
  - **Key Point:** *In the setting of severe TR, the Doppler envelope is often low velocity and early peaking because of high RA pressure. In this circumstance, it is difficult to estimate mean RAP and therefore accurately report PASP.*
  ---

PA end-diastolic pressure can be estimated using the PR jet (obtainable in the parasternal short axis at the level of the AoV). The end velocity of the PR jet represents the end-diastolic gradient between the PA and the RV (Fig. 5-7).
- PA end-diastolic pressure – RV end-diastolic pressure = $4 \times$ (end velocity of PR jet)$^2$

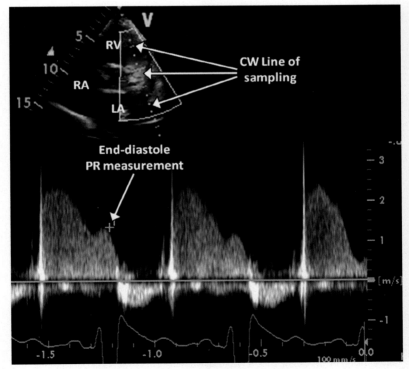

**Figure 5-7.** Continuous-wave Doppler across the pulmonic valve demonstrating estimation of the pulmonary end-diastolic pressure from the end-diastolic velocity of the PR jet.

- **PA end-diastolic pressure** $\approx 4 \times$ **(end velocity of PR jet)$^2$ + RA pressure**
- **Normal PA end-diastolic pressure <15 mmHg**
- **Mean PA pressure can be estimated using either (1) the RV outflow tract acceleration time or (2) the peak PR velocity.** For the RVOT acceleration time, PW Doppler 1 to 2 mm proximal to PV in parasternal short axis at level of AoV. **Closing click should be present but not opening click.** RVOT acceleration time = time to peak of RVOT outflow PW Doppler (Fig. 5-8).
  - **(1) Mean PA pressure $\approx 80 - \frac{1}{2} \times$ RVOT acceleration time**
  - In cases of very elevated PA pressures, a mid-systolic notch can be seen in the RVOT outflow Dopper jet, due to early transient closure of the PV.
  - **(2) Mean PA pressure $\approx 4 \times$ (peak velocity of PR jet)$^2$ + RA pressure**
  - **Normal mean PA pressure ≤25 mmHg**

---

- **Key Point:** *When measuring Doppler acquired gradients, ensure that the cardiac rhythm is regular. If the rhythm is irregular, average measurements from at least 5 to 10 cardiac cycles.*

---

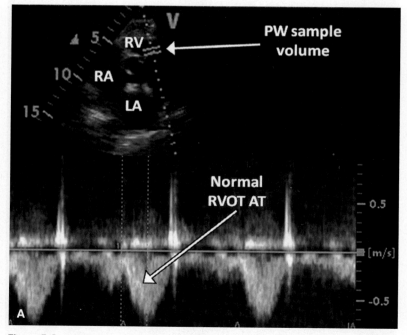

**Figure 5-8.** Pulsed-wave Doppler of the RVOT with correct positioning of the sample volume so that only the closing click is recorded. Measurement of the RVOT acceleration time from onset to peak velocity allows estimation of mean PA pressure. **(A)** Normal RVOT acceleration time (AT).

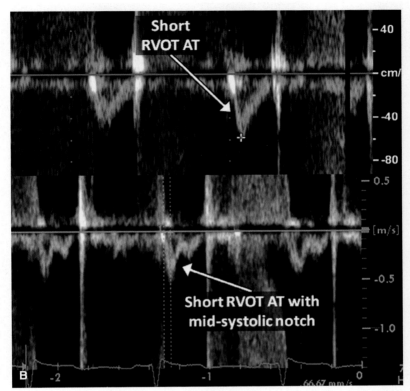

**Figure 5-8.** *(Continued)* **(B)** Short RVOT acceleration time and mid-systolic notching suggesting elevation of mean PA pressure.

## Estimating Mean RA Pressure

- The IVC is a highly compliant vessel that acts as a reservoir for the right atrium. The size and respiratory variation of this vessel thus reflects right-sided hemodynamics and can be used to estimate mean RA pressure.
- Measure the IVC **½ to 3 cm from RA junction** in the subcostal view during quiet respiration and after "sniff" maneuver. M-mode can be placed on the IVC for more accurate quantification (Fig. 5-9).
  - **IVC ≤2.1 cm with respiratory variation >50% = 0 to 5 mmHg**
  - **IVC >2.1 cm with respiratory variation <50% = 10 to 20 mmHg**
  - **IVC changes not fitting the above are categorized by an intermediate RA pressure value of 5 to 10 mmHg. Alternative methods for RA pressure estimation should also be assessed.**

---

- **Key Point:** *In assessing IVC diameter, ensure that the reduction in caliber, suggesting normal RA pressure, is due to changes with respiration rather than translational movement secondary to probe or patient motion.*

---

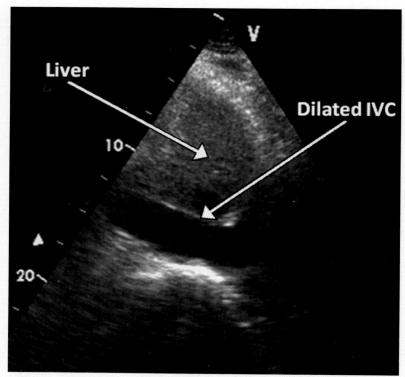

**Figure 5-9.** Subcostal image showing dilated IVC. Measurement of the IVC diameter should be taken close to the RA and IVC junction.

- Hepatic Doppler can be used to corroborate IVC findings. Systolic flow is greater than diastolic flow when mean RA pressure is normal. In the absence of severe TR, blunting of systolic flow suggests elevated mean RA pressure (Fig. 5-10).
- IVC dilatation is not always a reliable estimate of elevated RA pressure in young patients, mechanically ventilated patients, and patients with prominent eustachian valves. In these cases, an alternative estimation of RA pressure should be obtained using Doppler imaging of the TV.
  - Using the TV inflow (PW Doppler at tips of TV), determine the early tricuspid inflow velocity (E-wave). Using tissue Doppler imaging of the lateral TV annulus, determine the early tricuspid annular velocity (e'-wave).
  - **E/e' > 6 indicates a mean RA pressure >10 mmHg.**

### Exceptions to the Rule: When the Doppler Does not Agree with the Cardiac Catheterization

There are several explanations as to why a Doppler-derived estimation of right-sided pressures may be inconsistent with invasive pressure measurements.

- If the transducer is **not parallel** to the flow of the TR jet, the peak velocity of the jet will be reduced and lead to an underestimation of the PASP (see Chapter 1).

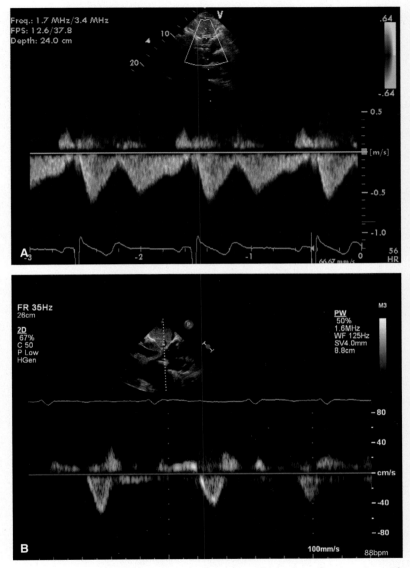

Figure 5-10. (A) Normal hepatic Doppler showing systolic dominant flow in patient with normal RA pressure. (B) Abnormal hepatic Doppler showing systolic blunting and diastolic dominant flow in patient with elevated RA pressure and severe pulmonary hypertension.

Also in TR Doppler envelopes where spectral broadening is present, not measuring the modal velocity may result in overestimation of PASP. Note any error in velocity measurement is "**squared**" using the modified Bernoulli equation.

- Incorrectly estimating mean RA pressure from the **IVC** can lead to under- or over-estimation of pulmonary pressures.
- Inability to accurately estimate mean RA pressure in the setting of severe TR.
- Accidently capturing the MR jet instead of the TR jet can lead to a gross overestimation of PA pressures. In cases where pulmonary pressures are near systemic pressures, it is imperative to ensure that the TR and not MR jet Doppler envelope is measured. The jet of TR will always be **longer** in duration than MR (due to longer isovolumic relaxation and contraction times) and will demonstrate respiratory variation.

**Using multiple methods to confirm your findings will improve your accuracy and consistency in reporting pulmonary pressures.** With the exception of acute pulmonary embolism, a high velocity TR jet should be accompanied by a short RVOT acceleration time. Additional findings to support a diagnosis of pulmonary hypertension should also be found (e.g., RV hypertrophy or enlargement, "D-shaped" LV, PA enlargement, IVC and coronary sinus dilatation, blunted systolic hepatic flow, interatrial septum bowed toward LA).

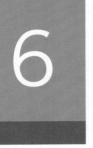

# 6 Stress Testing for Ischemia and Viability

Daniel H. Cooper and Thomas K. Kurian

## KEY POINTS

- Echocardiographic stress testing is a sensitive and specific modality for detecting the presence of stress-induced ischemia in appropriately selected patients.
- Ischemia manifests as regional wall motion abnormalities and changes in **myocardial thickening** during stress.
- Exercise echocardiography yields additional prognostic information and is preferred to pharmacologic stress testing.
- Causes of **false negative** results include: Failure to reach target heart rate, delayed peak stress image acquisition, single-vessel disease especially involving the circumflex artery, anti-anginal/beta-blocker use before testing.
- Causes of **false positive** results include: HTN, LVH, coronary spasm, paradoxical septal motion secondary to conduction abnormality (LBBB, pacing).
- To avoid these pitfalls, recognize the importance of achieving an adequate level of stress (>85% MPHR), timely image acquisition (<60 s for exercise echo protocols), and **confirming wall motion abnormalities in multiple views**.
- Dobutamine stress echocardiography can be utilized to confirm myocardial viability by noting the presence of a **biphasic response** to increasing rates of dobutamine infusion.

## General Principles

- The use of stress echocardiography for detection of ischemia is based on the principles outlined by the ischemic cascade (see Fig. 6-1).
- Impaired myocardial perfusion due to coronary artery disease (CAD) leads to a progression of manifestations during exercise or pharmacologic stress that ultimately results in regional or global wall motion or thickening abnormalities.
- The goal is to determine whether ischemia is present or, if there are baseline wall motion abnormalities and reduced LVEF, if there is viable myocardium and LV contractile reserve.
- Obtaining an adequate level of stress is vital to maintaining the modality's sensitivity for detecting CAD.
  - Achieving 85% of the maximally predicted heart rate (MPHR = 220 − Age) improves sensitivity greatly.
  - However, if changes consistent with ischemia are detected at lower (submaximal) levels of stress, this improves specificity of the result.

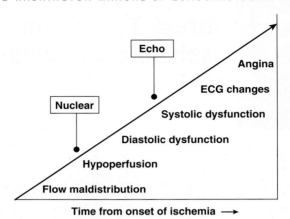

**Figure 6-1.** Ischemic cascade showing at what stage stress echocardiography and nuclear stress detect changes. (Schinkel AFL, Bax JJ, Geleijnse ML, et al. Noninvasive evaluation of ischaemic heart disease: myocardial perfusion imaging or stress echocardiography? *Eur Heart J.* 2003;24:789–800, by permission of Oxford University Press.)

- Continuous patient monitoring by medical staff is required, including frequent symptom inquires, continuous ECG, and intermittent BP measurement.
  - Crash carts, stocked with resuscitation equipment and medications, should be available.
- Risk of MI/Death ~1/2500

## Anatomy

- Stress echocardiography typically focuses on images obtained in the apical (four- and two-chamber) and parasternal (short- and long-axis) views, allowing for observation of all myocardial segments.
- Knowledge of the **typical distribution of coronary artery blood flow** to the various myocardial segments is vital. It allows:
  - Confirmation in multiple views of suspected lesions, especially when image quality in one view is suboptimal.
  - Correlation of findings to specific location(s) of coronary artery stenosis (Fig. 6-2).
    - **LAD:** Anterior, anteroseptal, apex, +/− inferoapical (wrap-around LAD)
    - **Circumflex:** Anterolateral, inferolateral
    - **RCA:** Inferior, inferoseptal (basal, mid), +/− inferolateral (depending on dominance)
    - **Distal versus proximal:** A proximal LAD lesion; for example, will result in basal to distal wall motion abnormalities of the anteroseptum (septal perforators) and anterior wall (diagonal) whereas distal LAD disease will affect only the apex.

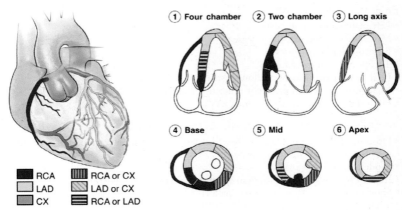

**Figure 6-2.** The standard echocardiographic views demonstrating the 17-segment model color-coded for typical coronary artery distribution. (Reprinted from Lang RM, Bierig M, Devereux RB, et al. Recommendations for Chamber Quantification: A Report from the American Society of Echocardiography's Guidelines and Standards Committee and the Chamber Quantification Writing Group, Developed in Conjunction with the European Association of Echocardiography, a Branch of the European Society of Cardiology. *JASE.* 2005; 18:1440–1463, with permission from Elsevier.)

## EXERCISE STRESS ECHOCARDIOGRAPHY

- In general, all exercise stress protocols involve staged increases in workload to increase myocardial oxygen demand. This is accomplished by treadmill or stationary bicycle exercise.
  - The Bruce protocol (most common) involves symptom-limited exercise on the treadmill where **grade and speed increases** every **3 minutes**.
  - METS (metabolic equivalents) are calculated automatically by the machine and is important to report as a prognostic indicator (<5 METS suggests poor prognosis if <65 years old).

### Absolute Contraindications

- Acute MI
- High-risk unstable angina
- Uncontrolled ventricular (VT) or supraventicular tachycardia (SVT)
- Severe arterial hypertension; systolic blood pressure (SBP) >200 mmHg and/or diastolic blood pressure (DBP) >110 mmHg
- Symptomatic severe aortic stenosis
- Uncontrolled, symptomatic congestive heart failure (CHF)
- Acute PE or pulmonary infarct
- Acute myocarditis or pericarditis
- Acute aortic dissection

### Relative Contraindications

- Left main coronary stenosis
- Moderate stenotic valvular disease
- Electrolyte abnormalities
- Tachy- or bradyarrhythmias
- HCM or other forms of outflow obstruction
- Mental or physical impairment inhibiting exercise
- High-degree atrioventricular block (AVB)

### Absolute Indications to Terminate Exercise Testing

- Drop in SBP >10 mmHg from baseline despite increase in workload, if accompanied by other evidence of ischemia
- Moderate to severe angina
- Increasing central nervous system symptoms (ataxia, near-syncope)
- Signs of poor perfusion (cyanosis, pallor)
- Technical difficulties in monitoring BP/ECG
- Patient's request
- Sustained VT
- ST elevation ≥1.0 mm in leads without Q waves (other than V1 or AVR)

### Relative Indications to Terminate Exercise Testing

- Drop in SBP >10 mmHg from baseline despite increase in workload, without other evidence of ischemia.
- ECG changes such as marked ST↓ (>2 mm, horizontal or downsloping) or marked axis shift
- Other arrhythmias (multifocal non-sustained VT, SVT, high-degree heart block, bradyarrythmia)
- Fatigue, shortness of breath, wheezing, leg cramps, claudication
- Increasing chest pain
- Hypertensive response (SBP >220 mmHg and/or DBP >115 mmHg)

## DOBUTAMINE STRESS ECHOCARDIOGRAPHY

- Pharmacologic stress is indicated in patients unable to exercise. Dobutamine is the most commonly utilized pharmacologic stress agent.
  - Dobutamine, like exercise, increases myocardial oxygen demand by augmenting contractility (positive inotropy), increasing heart rate (positive chronotropy), and elevating the blood pressure.
- Images are obtained at rest and at increasing doses of dobutamine infusion.
  - Typically, 4 to 5 three minute stages are utilized: 5, 10, 20, 30, 40 mcg/kg/min.
  - Atropine (0.2–0.4 mg every 2 minutes to a maximum of 2 mg) is commonly used to help achieve target heart rates, especially if patients have resting bradycardia or in the setting of beta-blockade. Use of this medication also reduces the occurrence of the Bezold–Jarisch reflex (profound vagal response) that may occur especially in the elderly (small LV cavity) and patients with hypovolemia.
- Side effects
  - Anxiety, nausea, headache, and palpitations from isolated premature beats are not uncommon.
  - Estimated risk for sustained ventricular arrhythmias or MI ~1/2000.

## Interpretation

*Baseline TTE*
- Particular attention should be given to **other possible causes of the symptoms** that prompted the ischemic evaluation. This is assessed from a baseline TTE performed prior to stress testing.
  - Specifically, new depressed LV function, pericardial tamponade, evidence of pulmonary embolism, severe aortic stenosis (AS) and aortic dissection should be excluded.
- In the absence of acute coronary syndrome (ACS), prior MI, or cardiomyopathy, wall motion and thickening should be normal on resting images in patients presenting with chest pain, even in the setting of significant CAD.
- However, be aware that regional wall motion abnormalities may be related to non-CAD causes. For example, "pseudodyskinesis" describes diastolic flattening of the inferior wall related to localized compression by the diaphragm. This is overcome during systole when the inferior wall becomes rounded giving the appearance of dyskinesis despite normal wall thickening. Pathologic causes of LV regional wall motion abnormalities include infiltrative disease (e.g., sarcoidosis), conduction abnormalities (e.g., left bundle branch block), post-cardiac surgical changes (paradoxical septal motion, myocardial patch repair), right heart abnormalities (e.g., volume or pressure overload), and stress-induced cardiomyopathy.

*Peak Stress TTE*
- Compare rest and stress **global and regional LV function in all available views** (parasternal short-axis, long-axis, apical four-chamber, apical two-chamber)
  - Wall thickening and movement is assessed in all myocardial segments.
  - Each of the 17 myocardial segments are graded by a five-point scale: Normal (1); hypokinetic, <30% wall thickening (2); akinetic, <10% wall thickening (3); dyskinetic, systolic outward movement (4); or aneurysmal, outwardly displaced segment in systole and diastole (5).
  - A wall motion score index (WMSI) can be calculated to quantify the extent of regional wall motion abnormalities.
  - WMSI = sum of wall motion scores/number of segments visualized (Normal = 1)
- Abnormal segments should be confirmed in **multiple views** to improve specificity.
  - For example, hypokinesis of the anteroseptal wall seen on the PLAX view should be confirmed on the PSAX view. In addition, are other myocardial segments subtended by the same coronary artery affected?
- **Recovery images** should be obtained to confirm resolution in patients with stress-induced wall motion abnormalities prior to discharge from the laboratory.

## False Results

- False negatives
  - Submaximal stress (<85% MPHR) is the most common cause.
  - Late image acquisition (>60 s) after peak exercise.
  - Single-vessel disease is more likely to be missed than multivessel because of the reduced extent of wall motion abnormalities seen.
  - Circumflex stenosis in particular is more commonly missed due to the relatively small myocardial territory involved.
  - Marked LVH and small LV cavity (increases the possibility of missing wall motion abnormality)
  - Beta-blocker/anti-anginal use

- False positives
  - Ischemia in the absence of epicardial CAD
    - Hypertensive response to stress
    - LVH
    - Microvascular disease (e.g., diabetes)
    - Coronary spasm (especially seen with dobutamine)
  - Non-ischemic causes of stress-induced wall motion abnormalities
    - Non-ischemic cardiomyopathy
    - Long-standing hypertension
    - Paradoxical septal motion (e.g., left bundle branch block)

## Prognosis

- Negative predictive value (NPV)
  - Event-free survival (MI or death) at three years ~99% if negative exercise stress echocardiogram.
  - Patients with a negative pharmacologic stress echocardiogram tend to have a slightly higher event rate, presumably secondary to the inability to exercise selecting for a "sicker" patient population.
- Cardiac risk increases incrementally with abnormal findings on a stress echocardiogram. In general, the following factors suggest a worse prognosis:
  - Ischemia at low thresholds (exercise or pharmacologic)
  - Extensive (4 to 5 myocardial segments) ischemia
  - Failure to reduce LV or worse, an increase in cavity size at peak exercise

## Other Considerations

- Stress echocardiography versus myocardial perfusion imaging
  - In general, stress echocardiography offers better specificity and slightly reduced sensitivity than myocardial perfusion imaging. This reduction in sensitivity is mostly related to single-vessel (especially circumflex artery) disease.
  - Overall, accounting for slight differences in sensitivity and specificity, both modalities offer similar accuracy and prognostic implications for patients presenting with symptoms and an intermediate risk of CAD.
- Given the importance of achieving target heart rate, beta-blockers should typically be held the day of the procedure.
  - However, for patients with known CAD, some physicians prefer to continue medical therapy to help gauge adequacy of treatment.
- Given the importance of endocardial border definition, echocardiographic contrast should be considered in patients with poorly defined myocardial segments.

# STRESS TESTING FOR MYOCARDIAL VIABILITY

## General Principles

- The role of stress echocardiography in detecting myocardial viability involves the demonstration of myocardial contractile reserve.
- Myocardial thickening is impaired when 20% or more of the wall is affected by ischemia or infarction.
- Therefore despite resting regional akinesis, a large proportion of myocardium may be viable and when stimulated allow normal myocardial thickening.

- "Hibernating" myocardium describes akinesis secondary to chronic ischemia with the important prognostic implication that coronary revascularization will restore normal myocardial function.
- Akinetic segments that are thinned and fibrotic (echogenic) at rest are less likely to be viable.
- Response of akinetic segments to increasing dobutamine infusion allows differentiation of viable myocardium from myocardial scar.

## Protocol

- Initial infusion typically begins at 2.5 mcg/kg/min with staged increases in dose to 5, 7.5, 10, and 20 mcg/kg/min.
- 40 mcg/kg/min can be utilized if improvement is sustained at 20 to 30 mcg/kg/min.
- Transthoracic echocardiographic images are obtained at rest and with each stage of dobutamine infusion. This includes PSAX, PLAX, A4C, and A2C views.
- The test should be terminated if there is absence of functional improvement or worsening of function during infusion.
- **Medical staff awareness of arrhythmia risk and careful monitoring for arrhythmias should be a particular focus during these studies.**
- By definition, these patients have some degree of scar-based structural heart disease that may serve as substrate for reentrant ventricular arrhythmias, particularly during dobutamine infusion.

## Interpretation

- Rest images
  - Baseline wall thickness and motion abnormalities should be noted in each segment.
- Bright, thinned-out (<0.6 cm) segments are consistent with nonviable scar that would not respond to revascularization.
  - Evidence of comorbid valvular heart disease should be carefully evaluated as it may change surgical risk and approach.
- Stress images
  - Evidence of functional improvement in affected segments with stress should be gauged.
  - Definition of viability: Improvement by one grade or more (i.e., akinetic → hypokinetic, normal, or hyperkinetic) in two or more myocardial segments.
  - Potential responses of affected segments to dobutamine infusion are shown in Table 6-1.

| TABLE 6-1 | Characteristic Echocardiographic Responses to Dobutamine Infusion to Determine the Etiology of Regional Akinesis | | | |
|---|---|---|---|---|
| Patient | Low-dose dobutamine | Peak-dose dobutamine | Viable myocardium | Critical coronary stenosis |
| Myocardial scar/ infarction | No increase | No increase | No | Yes |
| Hibernating myo-cardium | Increase | Decrease | Yes | Yes |
| Non-ischemic cardiomyopathy | Increase | Increase | Yes | No |

- DSE for viability is most reliable (specific) when a "biphasic response" is noted (i.e., improved myocardial thickening at low-dose dobutamine that worsens at high-dose dobutamine infusion).
- Worsening LV dysfunction with dobutamine infusion suggests non-viable myocardium (poor prognosis) and the test should be stopped.

## Other Considerations

- **Beta-blocade can limit the ability to detect viable segments.** If limited viability is detected on beta-blockers, then consideration should be given to repeating the test without beta-blockade.

# 7 Ischemic Heart Disease and Complications of Myocardial Infarction

Michael Yeung

## HIGH-YIELD FINDINGS

- Echocardiography is useful in the evaluation of acute chest pain by assessing possible wall motion abnormalities to identify areas of possible ischemia, as well as ruling out other acute causes of chest pain such as aortic dissection and pulmonary embolism.
- Quick calculation of stroke volume (SV) may provide additional information in the unstable patient

$$SV = CSA_{LVOT} \times VTI_{LVOT}$$

- Color flow Doppler and agitated saline are helpful in the localization of ventricular septal rupture (VSR).
- Presence of a pericardial effusion during or after a myocardial infarction (MI) is suspicious for left ventricular wall rupture.
- The posteromedial papillary muscle is often affected in acute ischemic MR, given its single coronary supply from the posterior descending artery.
- Assessment of the etiology and severity of acute MR may require TEE evaluation.
- A neck diameter to maximal aneurysmal diameter ratio of <0.5 suggests pseudoaneurysm.

## EVALUATION OF CHEST PAIN SYNDROME IN THE ACUTE SETTING

- In the acute setting, the rapid detection of new wall motion abnormalities as well as mechanical conditions allows echocardiography to play an integral part in the evaluation of chest pain syndrome. In addition, the screening of other critical mediastinal entities such as aortic dissection, pulmonary embolism, and pericarditis makes echocardiography an essential diagnostic tool in the emergency room.
- The previously discussed ischemic cascade (see Chapter 6) outlines the progression of reduced coronary flow and the ability of different diagnostic modalities to accurately detect its clinical manifestations. Echocardiography allows for the early detection of impaired myocardial relaxation even prior to the appearance of reduced systolic endocardial thickening.

- **Key Point:** *The presence of ischemia can be detected by visualizing:*
  - (1) *A lack of endocardial wall thickening (<40%) during systole as well as appearance of new regional wall motion abnormalities.*
  - (2) *A delay in the timing of endocardial thickening (usually completed within the first half of systole) leading to* **tardokinesis** *and* **post-systolic thickening**.

Infarct can be differentiated from regions of ischemia by areas of akinetic, thinned-out myocardium.

- Review of the ECG before obtaining the echocardiogram is important in order to localize and correlate the affected area. If the patient has a history of prior infarct, access to a prior echocardiogram is helpful for comparison of regional and overall LV function.
- Contrast agents have greatly improved the echocardiographic diagnostic accuracy of MI in the acute setting by enhancing the detection of regional wall motion abnormalities as well as endocardial thickening.
- For further discussion on coronary anatomy and regional distribution, please refer to Chapter 6.

## MECHANICAL COMPLICATIONS OF ACUTE MYOCARDIAL INFARCTION

- Recurrent chest pain after MI should prompt suspicion and evaluation of recurrent ischemia, post-MI pericarditis, pericardial effusion, aortic dissection, or left ventricular rupture.
- Cardiogenic shock after MI can be the result of right ventricular dysfunction, left ventricular dysfunction, acute MR due to papillary muscle rupture and tamponade due to LV rupture. Right-sided dysfunction can be differentiated clinically from left-sided dysfunction by the presence of marked neck vein distension, peripheral edema and the conspicuous absence of pulmonary edema.
- A new holosystolic murmur after MI suggests either (1) ischemic mitral regurgitation due to papillary muscle dysfunction/rupture, (2) ischemic ventricular septal defect (VSD).

## LEFT VENTRICULAR DYSFUNCTION AND CARDIOGENIC SHOCK

- Echocardiography provides important quantitative information regarding chamber size, ventricular systolic and diastolic function, valvular hemodynamics and pericardial involvement.
- Stroke volume (SV) is an important indirect measurement that can assist in the evaluation of the patient's hemodynamic status ($CO = SV \times HR$).
- SV can be reliably calculated by measuring the cross sectional area ($CSA_{LVOT}$) and velocity time integral ($VTI_{LVOT}$) of the left ventricular outflow tract by PW Doppler ($SV = CSA_{LVOT} \times VTI_{LVOT}$).
- Mitral early blood flow (E) and annular (e′) velocities have been correlated with pulmonary capillary wedge pressure (PCWP). **A septal E/e′ ≥15 corresponds to a PCWP >20 mmHg** whereas an E/e′ ≤8 corresponds to a PCWP <15 mmHg. Intermediate E/e′ values of 9 to 14 are indeterminate for elevated PCWP and other factors should be evaluated (e.g., left atrial enlargement, presence of elevated pulmonary artery systolic pressure) (see Chapter 4).

## VENTRICULAR SEPTAL DEFECT

- VSD markedly increases risk of mortality and occurs within the first 3 to 6 days of MI.

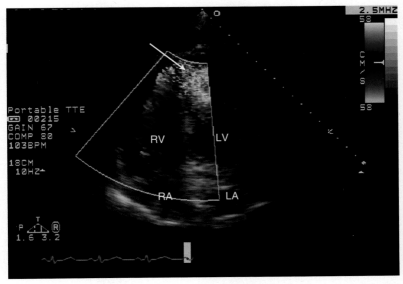

Figure 7-1. An apical four-chamber view with color Doppler showing a communication between the left and right ventricles in this apical VSD (*arrow*).

- Risk factors include age (>65 years), hypertension, female gender, first infarction, and single-vessel coronary disease. Its classic presentation is recurrent chest pain and hypotension several days after MI along with the presence of a new harsh pansystolic murmur and thrill in about 50% of the patients.
- The left anterior descending and right coronary arteries are most commonly implicated in the development of VSD. Anatomically, the left anterior descending artery supplies the apical portion of the ventricular septum, while the right coronary artery gives rise to the posterior septal perforators that supply the basal inferoseptal wall (see Figs. 7-1 and 7-2).
- VSDs may be simple or complex; with the latter often being associated with multiple areas as well as different dissection planes that track along the myocardium in a serpiginous fashion.
- The use of color flow Doppler is essential to identify the location of the left-to-right shunt. Off-axis views may be needed to better localize the rupture.
- The two most common locations are **inferoseptal** and **anteroapical walls.**
- Additional evaluation for worsening pulmonary hypertension, and left and right ventricular function is important for prognosis.
- Percutaneous closure is feasible in simple, apical VSDs.

> • **Key Point:** *Any localized areas of color disturbance or turbulence near the interventricular septum should be thoroughly investigated with off-axis imaging and spectral Doppler.*

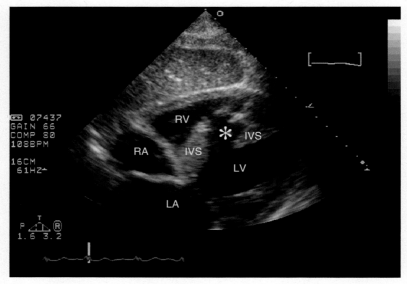

**Figure 7-2.** A subcostal view showing a complex, serpiginous VSD (*) in the interventricular septum (IVS).

## LEFT VENTRICULAR FREE WALL RUPTURE

- Cardiac free wall rupture is often a catastrophic event and approximately 40% of left ventricular free wall ruptures occur in the first day and 85% within the first week of the MI. High clinical suspicion by a rapidly deteriorating hemodynamic status after MI should prompt evaluation for myocardial rupture and transmutation MI, often in the anterior location.
- Predisposing factors include female gender, elderly (>65 years old), as well as single coronary disease (often total occlusion), anterior location, and transmural MI. Unsuccessful reperfusion and the delayed use of thrombolytics have also been associated with a higher incidence of free wall ruptures.
- Effusions are common in the setting of MI (up to 25% in acute setting). However, an expanding pericardial effusion with considerable wall thinning along the infarct region should raise suspicion of a left ventricular wall rupture. In addition, fibrinous echodensities in the pericardial space may be related to the presence of blood. Color flow Doppler increases the diagnostic yield and may help localize the site of myocardial tear (see Figs. 7-3 and 7-4).

## PAPILLARY MUSCLE RUPTURE AND ISCHEMIC MITRAL REGURGITATION

- Ischemic mitral regurgitation (IMR) may complicate MI classically presenting in the acute setting as sudden onset of hypotension and pulmonary edema, predominantly affecting the right upper lobe of the lung.

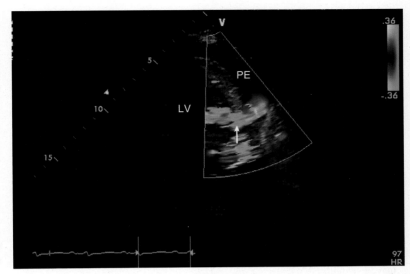

**Figure 7-3.** Apical four chamber with color flow Doppler. Color Doppler is instrumental in delineating the region of free wall rupture, which in this case is in the anterolateral wall (*arrow*). Notice the prominent pericardial effusion present (PE).

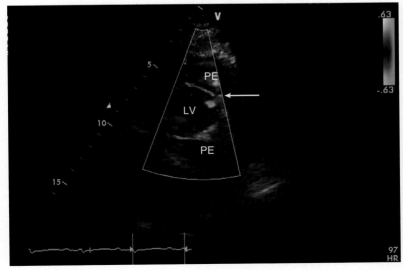

**Figure 7-4.** Short-axis view with color flow Doppler of LV wall rupture (*arrow*).

- In IMR, by definition, the mitral valve leaflets and subvalvular apparatus are **normal**. It is **adjacent myocardial ischemia, infarction and remodeling** surrounding the valve that leads to IMR.
- IMR; therefore, most commonly refers to tethering of the posterior mitral leaflet secondary to malpositioning and/or of the posteromedial papillary muscle (PMP) as a result of myocardial akinesis +/− remodeling. Less commonly papillary muscle rupture may occur in the setting of acute MI. The PMP is most commonly affected, because of a single arterial supply (right coronary or left circumflex artery depending on dominance). In contrast, the anterior–lateral papillary muscle (ALP) shares a dual supply from the left anterior descending and left circumflex arteries (see Figs. 7-5 and 7-6).
- In the setting of acute MI and MR, special attention should be paid not only to the severity of the MR, but also to the presence of abnormal leaflet motion (prolapse or flail). Acute IMR is suspected when the MR jet is eccentric, brief in duration (because of rapid rise in LA pressure) in the presence of a hyperdynamic LV and normal sized LA. The mitral E velocity is typically tall.
- Echocardiographic features differentiating acute IMR from chronic regurgitation include normal left heart and mitral annular sizes.
- Highly eccentric MR may be difficult to appreciate qualitatively or quantify by standard echocardiographic methods and higher resolution visualization by TEE may be helpful.
- Increased mortality has been associated with IMR than non-ischemic causes of MR and this is reflected in lower reference values used for severe MR of ischemic etiology (effective regurgitant orifice area $\geq 20$ mm$^2$, regurgitant volume $\geq 30$ mL).

---

- **Key Point:** *Severity of IMR may be visually underestimated because of eccentricity of jet and high LA pressure influencing jet size. Evaluation of leaflet motion for severe prolapse or flail segments is therefore critical for considering this diagnosis.*

---

## PERICARDIAL EFFUSION

- Small, uncomplicated pericardial effusions are common in transmural infarction and are usually transient in nature. These effusions result from inflammation of the epicardial wall and rarely result in tamponade.
- Large pericardial effusions after MI should raise the suspicion of ventricular free wall rupture, especially if the effusion appears to be hemorrhagic with thrombi or fibrinous material present in the pericardial space.
- Dressler's syndrome is a clinical entity that occurs 6 weeks to 3 months after MI. It is due to pericardial inflammation leading to reproducible chest pain and diffuses ST segment elevations on ECG. This inflammatory process results in increased permeability of the pericardium and subsequent accumulation of pericardial fluid.

---

- **Key Point:** *The subcostal view is usually best to visualize the full extent of a pericardial effusion especially if loculations and hematoma are present.*

---

## ACUTE DYNAMIC LEFT VENTRICULAR OUTFLOW TRACT OBSTRUCTION

- Acute dynamic LVOT obstruction is primarily seen in elderly females who present with an anterior MI. They often have a history of long-standing hypertension

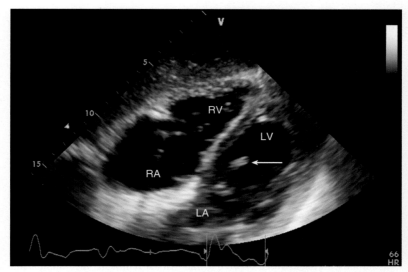

**Figure 7-5.** Modified subcostal view. A patient presenting with an inferior myocardial infarction and unexplained hypotension. An ovoid mass attached to the mitral valve chordae tendinae (*arrow*) is part of the posterior medial papillary muscle that has ruptured.

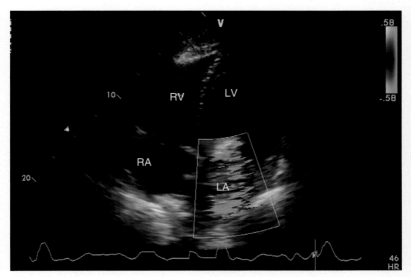

**Figure 7-6.** Same patient as Figure 7-5 with severe mitral regurgitation by color Doppler secondary to papillary muscle rupture seen in this apical four-chamber view.

with subsequent localized basal septal hypertrophy and small LV cavities. The obstruction develops as a result of the compensatory hyperdynamic function of the anteroseptal and inferolateral walls. This in turn leads to systolic anterior motion (SAM) of the mitral valve not unlike the classic presentation of hypertrophic cardiomyopathy, with corresponding LVOT obstruction and mitral valve regurgitation.

- Likewise, it may be present in ICU patients on inotropic therapy who are volume depleted.
- This entity has also been reported in up to 25% of patients with Takotsubo or stress-induced cardiomyopathy.

---

- **Key Point:** *Suspect acute dynamic LVOT obstruction in a patient with worsened hemodynamic status after initiation of inotropic therapy with no other obvious etiology.*

---

## LV PSEUDOANEURYSM

- LV pseudoaneurysm is the result of a rupture along the ventricular free wall with hemorrhage into the pericardial space that is self-contained by an organizing clot or thrombus. It occurs most often after MI, but may occur secondary to trauma or cardiac surgery.
- An abrupt acute angle is seen between the normal left ventricular myocardium and the aneurysmal region.
- A small, narrow neck connects the ventricular cavity with the walled off pericardial space.
- Pseudoaneurysms can be differentiated from true aneurysms by the following features:
  - The neck diameter to maximal aneurysmal diameter ratio is **<0.5.**
  - Color and spectral Doppler show **bidirectional** flow through the narrowed neck.
  - The identification of spontaneous echo contrast (stasis of blood) and **thrombus** in the pericardial space.
- In order of frequency, pseudoaneurysms occur most commonly in the inferior–posterior wall (Fig. 7-7), followed by the inferior–lateral and then apical walls (Fig. 7-8).
- Recognition of a pseudoaneurysm is critical because of a high risk of rupture and death.

## TAKOTSUBO SYNDROME

- Also referred to as stress-induced cardiomyopathy or apical ballooning syndrome.
- Classic presentation is that of a post-menopausal woman who has just experienced a psychological or physically **stressful event**.
- Often mimicking a true MI, this entity often presents with **ST segment elevation** as well as mildly elevated **positive biomarkers** for infarction. However, cardiac catheterization reveals **absence of obstructive coronary disease** to account for the patient's presentation.
- Although there are variants, the classic echocardiographic feature is **apical ballooning with a hypercontractile base,** giving an appearance similar to a Japanese octopus trap (Takotsubo).

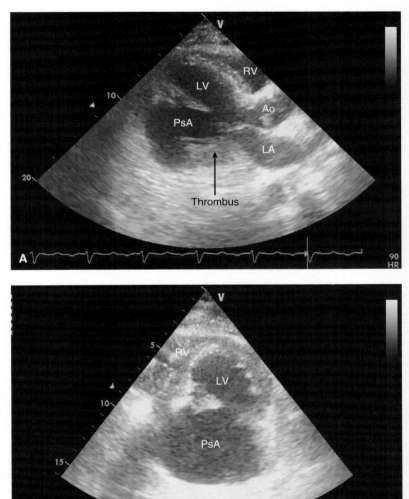

**Figure 7-7.** **(A)** PLAX and **(B)** PSAX views showing a large basal inferolateral pseudoaneurysm (PsA). Note thrombus within the pseudoaneurysm.

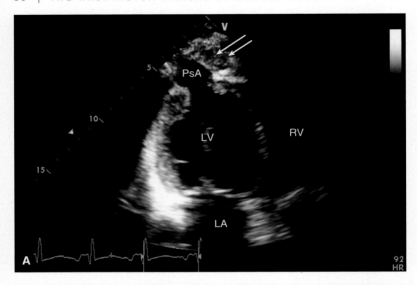

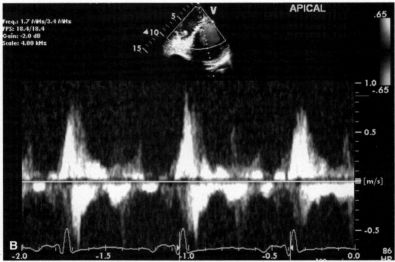

Figure 7-8. (A) An apical pseudoaneurysm (PsA) seen on an "off-axis" apical long-axis image. Note the narrow neck and thrombus in the pericardial space (*arrows*). (B) Spectral Doppler shows flow back and forward into the pseudoaneurysm.

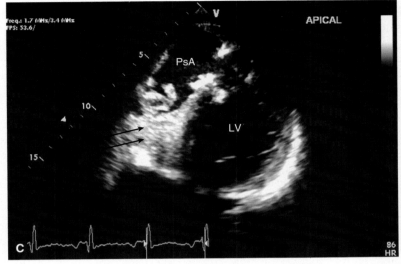

**Figure 7-8.** (*Continued*) (**C**) An off-axis apical two-chamber view shows the full extent of the pseudoaneurysm (PsA) and thrombus (*arrows*).

- Treatment is analogous to that of patients with heart failure and often resolves within days to months.
- Echocardiographic images of this syndrome are shown in Chapter 8.

## CHRONIC COMPLICATIONS OF ACUTE MYOCARDIAL INFARCTION

### Left Ventricular Aneurysm and Thrombus

- LV aneurysm is usually the result of a transmural infarction, causing thinning and remodeling of the ventricular wall.
- It occurs most frequently in the **apical** region but can occur anywhere.
- Complications of aneurysms include LV thrombus formation and ventricular arrhythmias.
- In general thrombi are dark and heterogeneous masses on echocardiography but may be bright if extensive fibrosis has taken place. They are almost always related to an akinetic or aneurysmal wall and may be laminar or pedunculated (prone to embolism).
- Contrast echocardiography has significantly increased detection of thrombi and also helps differentiate these masses from normal structures such as trabeculation or subvalvular structures.

---

- **Key Point:** *A foreshortened apical view is the most common reason why normal myocardial trabeculations may be mistaken for thrombus. This especially occurs when the heart is enlarged and the apex is aneurysmal causing trabeculations to appear prominent. Conversely, thrombus may be missed when the view is foreshortened. Use of a more lateral probe position and contrast for LV opacification will allow better visualization of the "true" LV apex and reduce these errors.*

---

## RIGHT VENTRICULAR DYSFUNCTION

- Right ventricular infarction occurs in up to 35% of patients who develop hypotension in the setting of inferior wall MI.
- On echocardiography, a dilated and hypokinetic right ventricle is seen. A dilated IVC with lack of respiratory variability and bowing of the interatrial septum toward the left atrium may also be seen due to elevated right atrial pressure.
- The apical RV may contract normally due to interaction with the LV and unaffected blood supply from the left anterior descending artery.
- Tricuspid regurgitation (TR) due to annular dilatation is usually present.
- Other characteristics of right-sided volume overload secondary to severe TR include flattening of the interventricular septum during diastole best seen on the parasternal short-axis view.
- In a patient with inferior MI presenting with sudden onset hypoxemia, suspect a patent foramen ovale (PFO) and the sudden development of right-to-left shunt due to elevated right-sided pressures from RV infarction. This can be detected by color Doppler, injection of agitated saline or transesophageal imaging.

# 8 Cardiomyopathies

Christopher L. Holley

## HIGH-YIELD FINDINGS

- *HCM* is characterized by LV hypertrophy in the absence of pressure overload; 35% of cases do not have any outflow obstruction
- Hypertrophic obstructive cardiomyopathy (*HOCM*) is a variant of HCM with outflow obstruction >30 mmHg; often with asymmetric septal hypertrophy (ASH), systolic anterior motion (SAM), and eccentric MR
- *DCM* is accompanied by both increased LV mass *and* volume; EF <55%; diastolic dysfunction is always present and central (functional) MR is common
- *RCM* involves restrictive filling without hypertrophy or dilation; it should prompt a thorough search for an underlying etiology, such as amyloid or other systemic illnesses
- *Arrhythmogenic right ventricular dysplasia (ARVD)* echocardiographic findings include RVOT diameter >30 mm and RV dysfunction in the presence of a normal LV. RV trabecular derangement is common
- *Takotsubo* cardiomyopathy is transient LV dysfunction with apical hypokinesis and basal hyperkinesis; *requires angiography to exclude significant CAD*
- *Non-compaction* is a developmental disorder with echocardiographic findings of abnormal LV trabeculation and cardiomyopathy

## KEY VIEWS

- *HCM:* PLAX to show abnormal septal or inferolateral wall thickness
- *HOCM:* PLAX (2D and M-mode) to look for ASH and SAM; A4C Doppler to demonstrate and localize LVOT gradient
- *DCM:* PLAX and A4C to show increased LV cavity diameter and volume; A4C Doppler to demonstrate diastolic dysfunction and look for MR
- RCM: A4C to assess restrictive filling by transmitral PW Doppler and low mitral annular tissue Doppler velocities
- *ARVD:* PLAX or PSAX to demonstrate RVOT enlargement; off-axis A4C to evaluate RV function and search for structural abnormalities
- *Takotsubo:* PLAX and A4C to show apical ballooning and hypercontractile basal segments
- *Non-compaction:* Apical and PSAX views *with contrast enhancement* to demonstrate abnormal LV trabeculation

The European Society of Cardiology uses this definition for cardiomyopathy: "A myocardial disorder in which the heart muscle is structurally and functionally abnormal, in the absence of coronary artery disease, hypertension, valvular disease, and congenital heart disease sufficient to cause the observed myocardial abnormality." (Elliott, P, et al. Classification of the cardiomyopathies: a position statement from the European Society Of Cardiology Working Group on Myocardial and Pericardial Diseases. *Eur Heart J.* 2008;29:270–276.) The five broad categories of cardiomyopathy are:

- Hypertrophic cardiomyopathy (HCM, including obstructive forms)
- Dilated cardiomyopathy (DCM)
- Arrhythmogenic right ventricular dysplasia (ARVD)
- Restrictive cardiomyopathy (RCM—see also Chapter 19)
- Other (including takotsubo and non-compaction cardiomyopathy)

## HYPERTROPHIC CARDIOMYOPATHY (HCM)

HCM is defined by the presence of increased ventricular wall thickness or mass in the absence of pressure overload. Such conditions that would otherwise lead to hypertrophy, such as hypertension and valvular heart disease (especially AS), must be excluded.

### Background

- Around 1:500 adults in the general population, men = women
- Important cause of sudden cardiac deaths in young adults
- *Majority* of patients do *not* have an outflow obstruction at rest
  - 35% of patients are not obstructed at rest *or* with provocation

### Echocardiographic Findings

- Left ventricular (LV) hypertrophy (increased mass), concentric or eccentric
  - Septal or inferolateral wall thickness >1.5 cm (PLAX or PSAX)
  - No LV dilatation
- HOCM: HCM with obstructive physiology
  - LVOT obstruction is **dynamic,** that is, increases with time during systole
  - **ASH** of the basal ventricular septum (see Fig. 8-1A)
  - **SAM** of the anterior mitral leaflet toward the septum
    - SAM:
      - Best seen in PLAX 2D or M-mode (see Fig. 8-1B)
      - May see mid-systolic contact of anterior leaflet with the septum in severe obstruction (Fig. 8-2).
      - LVOT obstruction may lead to mid-systolic closure or fluttering of the aortic valve because of reduced subvalvular pressure (Fig. 8-3A).
  - Eccentric **posteriorly directed, MR** jet secondary to SAM causing incomplete leaflet apposition (Fig. 8-3B)
    - As MR is mid to late peaking, it may be confused with the LVOT gradient.
    - A central or anterior jet should raise concern for intrinsic mitral valve pathology.
    - The MR jet peak velocity and systolic blood pressure (SBP) can be used to verify what the expected LVOT gradient should be and can be used as a "reality

check." In Figure 8-4, CW Doppler shows both the broader MR jet superimposed on the LVOT jet with measured gradients fitting with measured SBP.

- MR peak gradient = LVSP – LAP
∴ LVSP = MR peak gradient + LAP
- SBP = LVSP – LVOT gradient
∴ LVOT gradient = LVSP – SBP

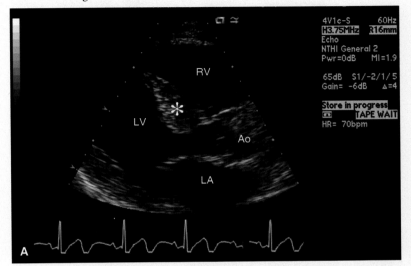

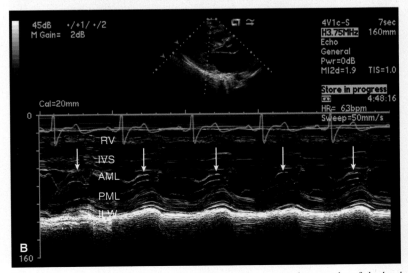

Figure 8-1. (A) Typical PLAX view for HOCM, with eccentric hypertrophy of the basal septum (*). (B) M-mode from the same view, demonstrates SAM of the MV anterior leaflet in systole (*arrows*).

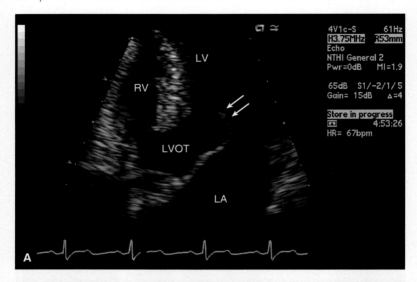

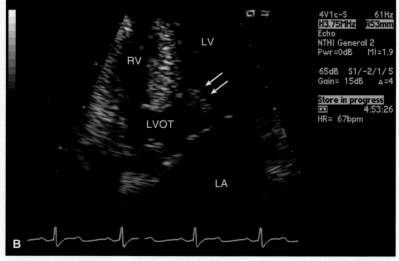

Figure 8-2. (A) A4C view of the MV during early systole and (B) mid-systole of the same beat, demonstrating systolic anterior motion of the valve (*arrows*). Note that in mid-systole, the MV contacts the septum suggestive of significant LVOT obstruction.

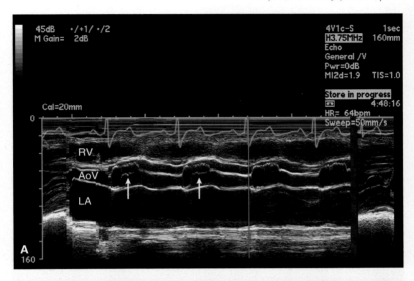

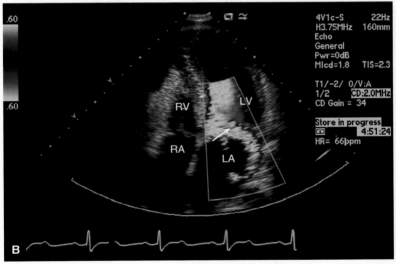

Figure 8-3. (A) Mid-systolic closure of the AoV due to dynamic LVOT obstruction (*arrows*). (B) Mid-systolic MR (*arrow*) with posteriorly directed jet due to SAM of the MV.

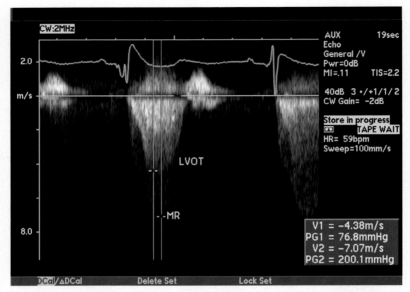

**Figure 8-4.** CW Doppler shows a higher velocity, slightly broader MR jet superimposed on a late-peaking LVOT jet. The patient's SBP ~120 mmHg at the time of the study serves as an additional indicator that the measured gradients were accurate (see text).

- Subaortic gradient: ≥30 mmHg (velocity ≥2.7 m/s)
  - CW Doppler will show **late-peaking Doppler** envelope ("broad-blade dagger" shape) due to dynamic nature of obstruction (Fig. 8-5A). Intracavitary LV gradients due to hyperdynamic LV function and small LV cavity are distinguished from LVOT gradients by having a "narrow-blade" and "pointy" late-peaking gradient (Fig. 8-5B). These both are in contrast to the early to mid-peaking Doppler envelope of fixed outflow obstruction (e.g., valvular AS, subaortic membrane) (Fig. 8-5C).
  - PW or high pulse repetition frequency (HPRF) Doppler must be used to identify the location of obstruction, which is often seen as turbulence on color Doppler (Fig. 8-6).
  - The gradient is influenced by both preload and afterload.
    - The gradient can be provoked/increased during echocardiography by Valsalva (decreases preload during strain phase), amyl nitrate inhalation (short acting vasodilator decreasing afterload), or inotropic medications (increased contractility).
    - The gradient should decrease with fluid bolus (increased preload) or vasoconstrictors (increased afterload).
- If an early-peaking subvalvular gradient that does not change with dynamic maneuvers is seen, TEE should be used to exclude a subaortic membrane (i.e., fixed subaortic obstruction that mimics AS).

---

- **Key Point:** *Evaluation of the Doppler profile and change in peak velocity with hemodynamic maneuvers helps differentiate dynamic LVOT obstruction of HOCM from fixed LVOT obstruction seen with subaortic membranes. Aortic insufficiency is also more typically seen with subaortic membranes whereas eccentric posterior mitral regurgitation is seen with HOCM.*

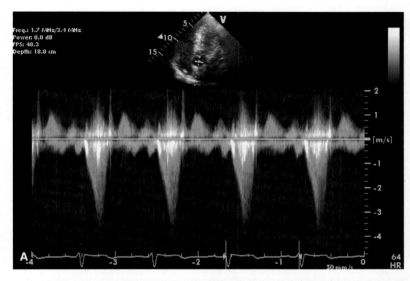

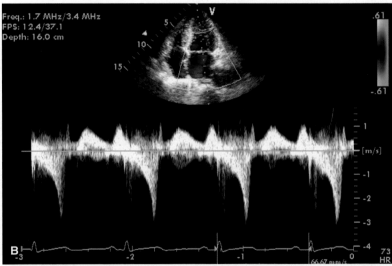

Figure 8-5. (A) Typical LVOT 'broad-blade' late-peaking gradient, (B) intracavitary 'narrow-blade' late-peaking gradient, and (C) fixed mid-peaking aortic stenosis gradient.(*continued*)

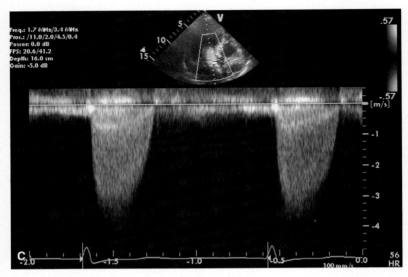

**Figure 8-5.** (*Continued*)

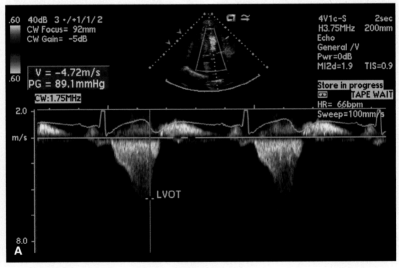

**Figure 8-6.** Panel A shows characteristic CW Doppler seen in HOCM.

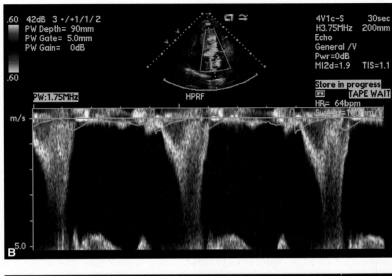

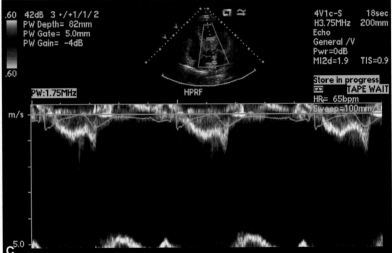

**Figure 8-6.** (*Continued*) Panels B and C show HPRF Doppler to localize the peak jet velocity (~4.7 m/s) as subvalvular (**B**) and not mid-cavity (**C**).

## DILATED CARDIOMYOPATHY (DCM)

Defined as LV dilatation and LV systolic dysfunction in the absence of abnormal loading conditions (e.g., hypertension, valvular disease) or coronary artery disease sufficient to cause global systolic impairment.

### Background

- ~25% of cases are familial (Western populations)
- Remaining cases are inflammatory/toxic/metabolic:
  - Myocarditis (infectious, toxic, immune-mediated)
  - Drugs/alcohol
  - Endocrine (e.g., thyroid)
  - Nutritional (e.g., thiamine/beriberi)
  - Tachycardia-mediated
  - Postpartum cardiomyopathy

### Echocardiographic Findings

- LV mass is uniformly increased (because the heart is simply bigger in overall dimensions) but wall thickness may be normal or reduced.
- Dilation (increased volumes) (Table 8-1 and Fig. 8-7A and B)
  - Increased sphericity (ratio of long/short LV axes; in these cases approaching 1.0 [normal = 1.5])
  - Mitral regurgitation is common as the mitral annulus dilates and papillary muscles are apically displaced leading to incomplete mitral valve coaptation; this is often termed "functional MR" (Fig. 8-7C).
- Impaired systolic function (Ejection fraction [EF] <55%)
  - Stroke volume may be preserved despite reduced EF, since LV diastolic volume is increased.
  - Look for mural thrombus in DCM with severe systolic dysfunction (IV contrast for LV opacification improves sensitivity).
- Impaired diastolic filling
  - Look for elevated E/e' as evidence of elevated mean left atrial pressure.

---

- **Key Point:** *DCM often affects all four cardiac chambers and so it is important to provide quantitative evaluation of size as well as function and filling pressures of LV and RV. Lateral probe position for image acquisition is important to provide non-foreshortened images because of cardiac enlargement.*

---

| TABLE 8-1 | Chamber Dimensions in Dilated Cardiomyopathy | | |
|---|---|---|---|
| | **LVIDd** | **LV diastolic** | **LV systolic** |
| ♀ | >5.3 cm | >104 mL | >49 mL |
| ♂ | >5.9 cm | >155 mL | >58 mL |

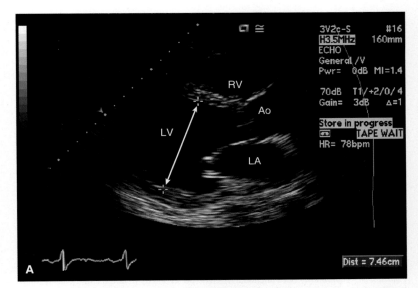

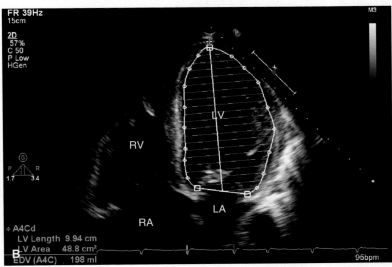

**Figure 8-7.** **(A)** Marked LV dilation, with LVIDd 7.46 cm. **(B)** Another patient with signifi-cant dilated cardiomyopathy and LV diastolic volume of 198 mL. See Table 8-1 for normal values. (*continued*)

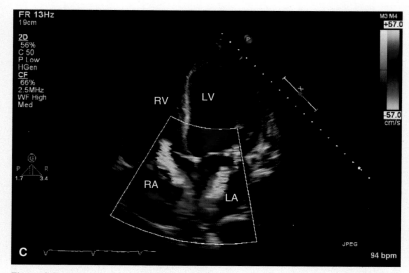

**Figure 8-7.** (*Continued*) **(C)** Functional MR and TR secondary to mitral and tricuspid annular dilatation.

## RESTRICTIVE CARDIOMYOPATHY (RCM)

RCM is defined by restrictive ventricular physiology in the presence of normal (or reduced) diastolic and systolic volumes. Strictly speaking, primary RCM is also defined by normal ventricular wall thickness, although secondary RCM can be caused by infiltrative disease (such as amyloid) that eventually leads to increased ventricular mass.

### Background

- Familial: Familial amyloidosis (e.g., transthyretin abnormality), hemochromatosis, glycogen storage disease, Fabry's (X-linked recessive lysosomal storage disease), and cardiac troponin mutations
- Non-familial: AL amyloid, endomyocardial fibrosis (including hypereosinophilic syndrome, drug-induced [e.g., serotonin]), carcinoid, radiation, chemotherapy (e.g., anthracyclines), scleroderma (see also Chapter 19 for cardiomyopathies caused by systemic illnesses)

### Echocardiographic Findings

- Restrictive diastolic filling, bi-atrial enlargement, normal systolic function, and no ventricular dilation.
- Restrictive mitral filling because of non-compliant LV.
  - E >100 cm/s, E/A >2, DT ≤160 ms, e′ <8 (septal), e′ <10 (lateral), E/e′ ≥15 (septal), E/e′ ≥12 (lateral), E/e′ ≥13 (average of septal and lateral) (see also Table 4-5 in Chapter 4).

- May be difficult to differentiate from constrictive pericarditis (an important distinction for patient management); however, in contrast to this disorder, restrictive cardiomyopathy tissue Dopper myocardial velocities are markedly reduced and hepatic Doppler flow reversals are most marked during *inspiration.*
- Myocardium may have an abnormal echogenic, sparkling appearance suggestive of infiltrative disease. If the interatrial septum is also affected this is suggestive of amyloidosis.
- 'Binary' appearance of LV myocardium in Fabry's disease with bright endocardium and myocardium with "clearing" of intervening subendocardium related to the compartmentalization and accumulation of glycosphingolipids in certain layers of the wall.
- Cardiac involvement in hyperesosinophilic syndrome involves eosinophilic infiltration of the myocardium causing necrosis and obliteration of the ventricular apex with thrombus. Endomyocardial fibrosis leads eventually to restrictive cardiomyopathy (Fig. 8-8).

---

- **Key Point:** *LV apical thrombus typically occurs in an area of akinesis or aneurysm formation. Hypereosinophilic syndrome is an example where thrombus can form without the presence of regional wall motion abnormalities.*

---

## ARRHYTHMOGENIC RIGHT VENTRICULAR DYSPLASIA (ARVD)

ARVD is defined by the presence of right ventricular dysfunction (global or regional), with or without LV disease, in the presence of histologic evidence for the disease and/or electrocardiographic abnormalities.

### Background
- Estimated prevalence 1:5,000

### Echocardiographic Findings
- Normal LV size and function
- Increased RV dimensions (Fig. 8-9A)
  - At the level of the RV outflow tract >30 mm, measured in diastole, PLAX or PSAX view
- Decreased RV function
- RV morphologic abnormalities also common
  - Trabecular derangement (see Fig. 8-8B)
  - Hyper-reflective moderator band
  - Saccular aneurysms

## TAKOTSUBO CARDIOMYOPATHY
See also Chapter 7.

### No Consensus Criteria, but Modified Mayo Clinic Criteria are Often Used:
- Transient hypokinesis, akinesis, or dyskinesis of mid to distal LV with apical involvement, in the setting of acute chest pain after physical or emotional stress (see Fig. 8-10).
- EKG abnormalities modest troponin elevation mimic acute coronary syndrome.

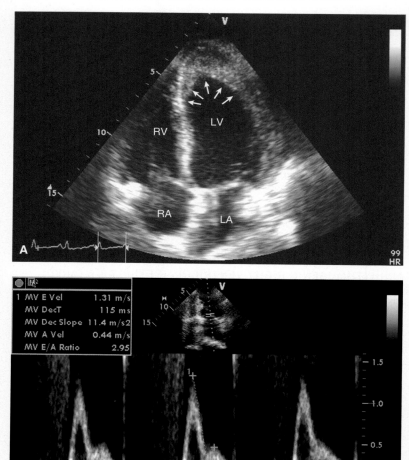

**Figure 8-8.** (A) A4C showing thrombus obliterating the LV apex (*arrows*) in patient with hypereosinophilic syndrome. No regional wall motion abnormalities were seen. (B) Restrictive mitral inflow Doppler with E/A ratio ≥2 and E wave deceleration time <160 msec.

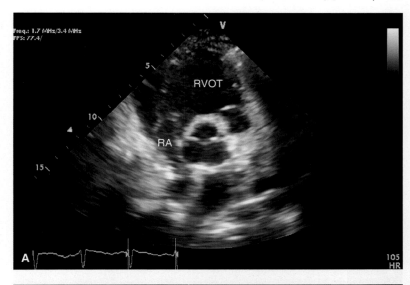

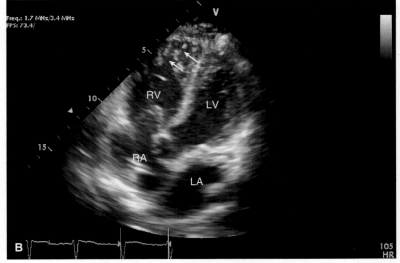

**Figure 8-9.** Patient with ARVD. **(A)** PSAX view with marked RVOT enlargement. **(B)** Off-axis A4C view demonstrates hypertrabeculation of the RV (*arrows*).

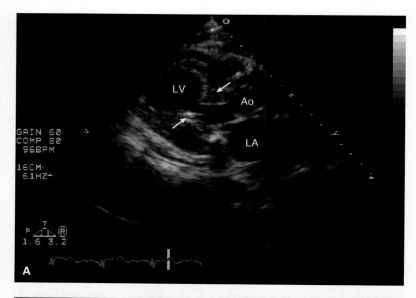

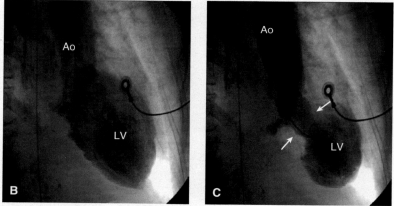

**Figure 8-10.** Patient with takotsubo cardiomyopathy. (**A**) PLAX during systole with marked basal hypercontractility and apical ballooning. Left ventriculograms from the same patient in diastole (**B**) and systole (**C**). The patient presented with pulmonary edema and cardiogenic shock in the setting of anterolateral ST elevation on electrocardiography. Peak serum troponin was 9 mcg/dL.

• No angiographic evidence of obstructive coronary disease or acute plaque rupture.
• No evidence of myocarditis or pheochromocytoma.

### Background
• Typical patient is postmenopausal woman with severe emotional (e.g., death of a spouse) or physical stress (e.g., surgery, severe pain, intracranial bleeding).
• Presents as acute chest pain and/or left heart failure that is reversible.

### Echocardiographic Findings
• ECHOCARDIOGRAPHY CANNOT DEFINITIVELY DIAGNOSE STRESS INDUCED CARDIOMYOPATHY! *Coronary artery disease must be excluded by angiography.*
• Takotsubo refers to the appearance of transient LV apical ballooning (Fig. 8-8).
    • Hypocontractile apical segments: Involving more than one coronary territory
    • Hypercontractile basal segments
• May affect both LV and RV.
• Myocardial involvement much greater than expected by cardiac enzyme elevation.
• Less commonly "Inverted" takotsubo pattern has also been described, with basal hypokinesis and apical sparing as well as a "Mid-LV" takotsubo pattern where there is mid-LV hypokinesis with sparing of the apex and basal segments.

> • **Key Point:** *This typical ventricular contractile pattern that resolves over time on echocardiography helps define the likelihood of this entity.*

## ISOLATED NON-COMPACTION OF THE LV

### Background
• **Prominent LV trabeculae, deep intertrabecular recesses,** thin epicardium, thick endocardium
• 0.014% incidence in series of consecutive echocardiograms
• Frequently familial, with evidence in up to 25% of asymptomatic relatives
    • Thought to be failure of normal LV trabecular compaction during fetal development (weeks 5 to 8)
• Clinical presentation: High prevalence of heart failure (systolic and diastolic), **thromboembolism,** and arrhythmia (Atrial fibrillation and ventricular tachycardia)

### Echocardiographic Findings:
• LV trabeculation with deep intertrabecular recesses (at least four seen in LV apical or PSAX views) (Fig. 8-11)
    • Primarily at the **apex** and mid **inferior/lateral** walls
    • Color flow Doppler demonstrates flow in the trabecular recesses
    • "Two-layered" ventricular wall, with **non-compacted endocardial layer ≥2× the thickness of compacted epicardial layer** (i.e., greater trabeculation than what would be expected in simple LV dilatation)
• No other cardiac abnormalities

> • **Key Point:** *The use of IV contrast for LV opacification increases sensitivity in detecting trabeculae, trabecular recesses and thrombi in LV non-compaction.*

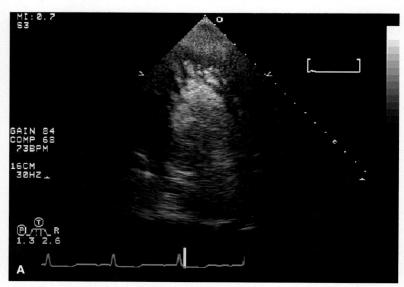

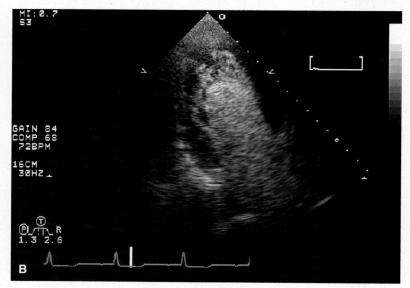

Figure 8-11. Non-compaction. Panels A and B show contrast-enhanced images of a non-compacted LV in the A4C and A2C views, respectively. Note the conspicuous trabeculation with deep intertrabecular recesses.

# Aortic Valve Disease

Brian R. Lindman and Suzanne V. Arnold

## HIGH-YIELD CONCEPTS

- *LVOT dimension* is a significant source of error when measuring AVA
- Make sure the numbers are internally consistent (AVA, gradients, LVEF)
- Subvalvular obstruction: Evaluate flow through the LVOT
- *Low-dose dobutamine test* is helpful in patients suspected of having severe AS in the setting of low flow, low gradients
- *LV size, shape, and function* are helpful in determining acute (normal LV size) versus chronic AR (dilated LV)

## KEY VIEWS

- *Parasternal long axis*—initial screening for AS severity (ability of valve to open, calcification) and AR severity (width of jet, LV dimensions); LVOT measurement
- *Parasternal short axis*—AoV morphology
- *Apical long axis and apical five-chamber views*—quantitative assessment of AS and AR: LVOT and AoV gradients, AR PHT using Doppler
- *Apical four chamber*—LV dimensions and LV function for AR chronicity
- *TEE*—higher resolution views for valve morphology, planimetry for AVA, AR severity

## SEVERITY OF AORTIC STENOSIS

See Table 9-1.

| TABLE 9-1 | Severity of Aortic Stenosis | | | |
|---|---|---|---|---|
| | Aortic sclerosis | Mild | Moderate | Severe |
| Aortic jet velocity (m/s) | ≤2.5 | 2.6–2.9 | 3.0–4.0 | >4.0 |
| Mean gradient (mmHg) | — | <20 (<30[a]) | 20–40[b] (30–50[a]) | >40[b] (>50[a]) |
| AVA (cm²) | — | >1.5 | 1.0–1.5 | <1.0 |
| Indexed AVA (cm²/m²) | — | >0.85 | 0.60–0.85 | <0.6 |
| Velocity ratio | — | >0.50 | 0.25–0.50 | <0.25 |

[a]ESC guidelines.

[b]AHA/ACC guidelines.

AVA, aortic valve area.

Adapted from Baumgartner H, Hung J, Bermejo J, et al. Echocardiographic assessment of valve stenosis: EAE/ASE recommendations for clinical practice. *J Am Soc Echocardiogr.* 2009;22(1):1–23, with permission from Elsevier.

## SEVERITY OF AORTIC REGURGITATION

See Table 9-2.

| TABLE 9-2 | Severity of Aortic Regurgitation | | | |
|---|---|---|---|---|
| | **Mild** | **Moderate** | | **Severe** |
| **Structural parameters** | | | | |
| LA size | Normal[a] | Normal or dilated | | Usually dilated[b] |
| Aortic leaflets | Normal or abnormal | Normal or abnormal | | Abnormal/flail, or wide coaptation defect |
| **Doppler parameters** | | | | |
| Jet width in LVOT—color flow[c] | Small in central jets | Intermediate | | Large in central jets; variable in eccentric jets |
| Jet density—CW | Incomplete or faint | Dense | | Dense |
| Jet deceleration rate—CW (PHT, ms)[d] | Slow >500 | Medium 500–200 | | Steep <200 |
| Diastolic flow reversal in descending aorta—PW | Brief, early diastolic reversal | Intermediate | | Prominent holodiastolic reversal |
| **Quantitative parameters[e]** | | | | |
| VC width, cm[c] | <0.3 | 0.3–0.60 | | >0.6 |
| Jet width/LVOT width, %[c] | <25 | 25–45 | 46–64 | ≥65 |
| Jet CSA/LVOT CSA,%[c] | <5 | 5–20 | 21–59 | ≥60 |
| R Vol, mL/beat | <30 | 30–44 | 45–59 | ≥60 |
| RF, % | <30 | 30–39 | 40–49 | ≥50 |
| EROA, cm[2] | <0.10 | 0.10–0.19 | 0.20–0.29 | ≥0.30 |

[a]Unless there are other reasons for LV dilation. Normal 2D measurements: LV minor axis ≤2.8 cm/m$^2$, LV end-diastolic volumes ≤82 mL/m$^2$.

[b]Exception: Would be acute AR, in which chambers have not had time to dilate.

[c]At a Nyquist limit of 50 to 60 cm/s.

[d]PHT is shortened with increasing LV diastolic pressure and vasodilator therapy, and may be lengthened in chronic adaptation to severe AR.

[e]Quantitative parameters can subclassify the moderate regurgitation group into mild-to-moderate and moderate-to-severe regurgitation as shown.

LA, left atrium; LVOT, left ventricular outflow tract; CW, continuous wave; PHT, pressure half-time; PW, pulsed wave; VC, vena contracta; CSA, cross-sectional area; R Vol, regurgitant volume; RF, regurgitant fraction; EROA, effective regurgitant orifice area.

Adapted from Baumgartner H, Hung J, Bermejo J, et al. Echocardiographic assessment of valve stenosis: EAE/ASE recommendations for clinical practice. *J Am Soc Echocardiogr.* 2009;22(1):1–23, with permission from Elsevier.

## ANATOMY

- **Leaflets**
  - The normal aortic valve (AoV) is trileaflet.
  - A bicuspid valve occurs in 1% to 2% of the population, unicuspid and quadricuspid valves are rare. The abnormal leaflet number may cause inherent valvular stenosis and regurgitation.
- **Annulus**
  - The leaflets form semi-lunar attachments at the annulus forming a "crown"-like interlocking of ventricular and arterial tissue.
  - They also attach at the sinotubular junction.
- **Sinuses of Valsalva**
  - As the proximal aortic root meets the left ventricular outlet there are three sinuses that bulge out and form the supporting structure for the corresponding aortic valve leaflets.
  - The sinuses and corresponding valve leaflet (or cusp) are named according to the origin of the coronary arteries.
  - Two sinuses give rise to coronary arteries (right and left) while the third, lying immediately adjacent to the mitral valve, does not (non).
- **Sinotubular junction**
  - The place where the superior portion of the sinuses narrows and joins the proximal tubular portion of the ascending aorta.

## AORTIC STENOSIS

- **Pathophysiology**

  The pathophysiology for aortic stenosis (AS) involves both the valve and the ventricular adaptation to the stenosis. Within the valve, there is growing evidence for an active biologic process that begins much like the formation of an atherosclerotic plaque and eventually leads to calcified bone formation.

---

Valvular obstruction → ↑Intraventricular pressure to maintain CO
↓
Ventricular wall hypertrophy to reduce wall stress
(Laplace's law: Wall stress = pressure × radius/2 × thickness)
↓
LVH → (1) ↓compliance, impaired passive filling, ↑preload dependence on atrial contraction;
(2) ↑LVEDP → subendocardial ischemia (↓myocardial perfusion pressure) and pulmonary congestion
↓
Progressive valvular obstruction, hypertrophy, fibrosis, and increasing wall stress
↓
Ischemia, arrhythmia, ↑filling pressure, ventricular dilation, contractile dysfunction, and ↓LVEF
↓
Angina, syncope, and dyspnea

---

- **Etiology and morphology**
See Table 9-3 and Figure 9-1.

| TABLE 9-3 | Etiology and Morphology of Aortic Valve Disease |
|---|---|
| **Etiology** | **Prevalence, presentation, and associated features** |
| **Normal** | • Asymptomatic |
| **Calcific/ Degenerative** | • Most common cause in the United States<br>• Presents in seventh to ninth decades (mean age mid-70s)<br>• Risk factors similar to CAD<br>• Calcification leading to stenosis affects both trileaflet and bicuspid valves |
| **Bicuspid** | • 1–2% of population (the most common congenital lesion)<br>• Presents in sixth to eighth decades (mean age mid-late 60s)<br>• More prone to endocarditis than trileaflet valves<br>• Associated with aortopathies (i.e., dissection, aneurysm, coarctation) |
| **Rheumatic** | • Most common cause worldwide, much less common in the United States<br>• Presents in third to fifth decades<br>• Almost always accompanied by mitral valve involvement |

Adapted from Zoghbi WA, Enriquez-Sarano M, Foster E, et al. Recommendations for evaluation of the severity of native valvular regurgitation with two-dimensional and Doppler echocardiography. *J Am Soc Echocardiogr.* 2003;16(7):777–802, with permission from Elsevier.

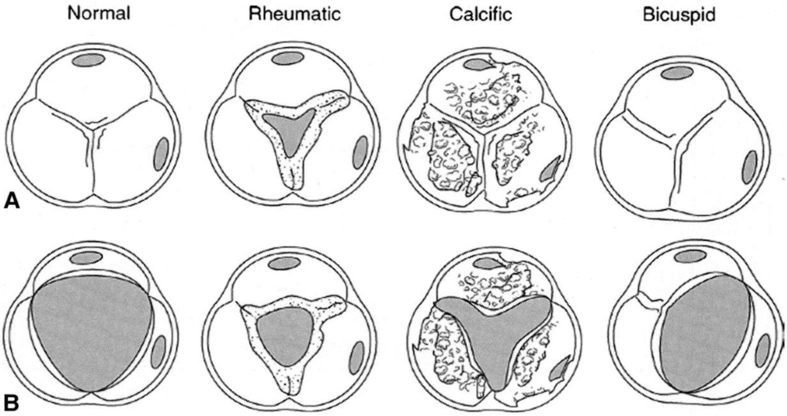

Figure 9-1. Typical appearance of aortic valve in diastole (row A) and systole (row B) suggestive of underlying etiology. (Adapted from C. Otto, *Principles of Echocardiography,* 2007.)

- **Echocardiographic assessment of AS**
  - **2D assessment**
    - ○ **Leaflets**
      - *Motion of the valve*
        - Aortic valve area (AVA) can be planimetered in the parasternal short-axis view—this is most often only possible in TEE studies using a side-by-side zoomed short-axis 2D image with corresponding color Doppler image to ensure that correct margins are drawn.
        - Ensure that your visual estimate of valve orifice area corresponds with other measurements; if, for example, the valve appears to open fairly well but measured gradients are considerably higher than you would expect, there may be a supra/subvalvular obstruction. Conversely if the valve appears calcified and stenotic; however, the recorded gradients are lower than expected consider: (1) Doppler acquisition not parallel to flow, (2) low flow, low gradient, reduced LVEF AS, (3) low flow, low gradient, normal LVEF AS (discussed later).
        - Eccentric closure, doming, and prolapse of the valve in the parasternal long-axis view suggest the presence of a bicuspid valve.

> - **Key Point:** *In the PLAX, the right coronary cusp (closest to RV) and typically the non-coronary cusp are seen. In the PSAX view the non-coronary cusp lies near the interatrial septum, the right coronary cusp near the RVOT and left near the LA. (Moving clockwise use pneumonic NoRmaL!)*

      - *Bicuspid aortic valves (BAVs)*—most commonly due to fusion of the right and left coronary cusps (~80%) or fusion of the right and non-coronary cusps (~20%); bicuspid valves have an elliptical orifice during systole; they can easily be mistaken for trileaflet valves during diastole, particularly when a raphe is present. Leaflet doming is present because of restricted leaflet motion. Valvular regurgitation is usually highly eccentric and posteriorly directed (Fig. 9-2E). There may be associated aortic abnormalities (dilation of aortic root, coarctation).
      - *Rheumatic aortic valve*—leaflet thickening and fusion affects the **tips** predominantly causing doming of the valve.
      - *Calcification*—the distribution and amount of calcification is important to note as it suggests an etiology and impacts prognosis. In senile calcific AS there is calcification of the **body** of the leaflets as well as the supporting aortic root.
    - ○ **Supravalvular or subvalvular obstruction**
      - *Subvalvular obstruction* can be *fixed* (e.g., subaortic membrane) or *dynamic* (e.g., hypertrophic cardiomyopathy with obstruction). A subaortic membrane is often seen best in the apical long-axis or apical five-chamber views and is usually a tunnel-shaped circumferential fibrous ring or a discrete fibrous ridge. There is often concomitant AR secondary to left ventricular outflow tract (LVOT) turbulence affecting the aortic valve. In contrast, a dynamic obstruction is usually caused by systolic anterior motion (SAM) of the anterior leaflet of the mitral valve being dragged into the LVOT during systole causing a late peaking gradient. Dynamic means that provocative maneuvers that alter preload or afterload will alter the gradient.
      - *Supravalvular obstruction* is an uncommon congenital condition and is best visualized in the high PLAX view.

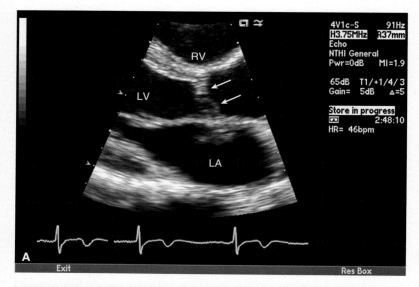

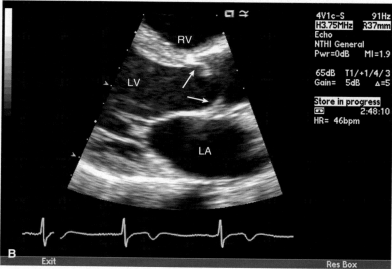

**Figure 9-2.** Movement of the aortic valve and the importance of assessing number of cusps in systole. Images taken from a patient with BAV. **A:** PLAX in diastole, aortic valve leaflets prolapse behind annular plane (*arrows*). **B:** PLAX in systole, doming of aortic valve leaflets signifying restricted motion (*arrows*).

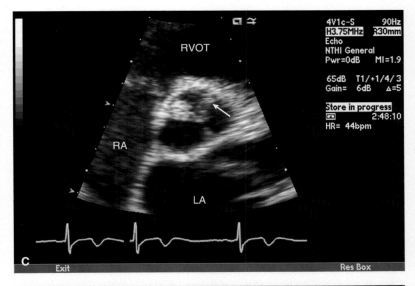

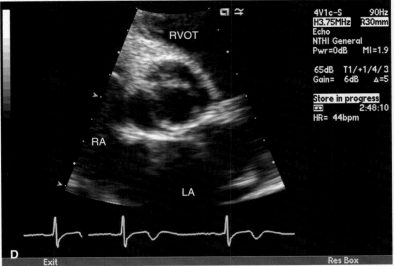

**Figure 9-2.** (*Continued*) **C:** PSAX in diastole, aortic valve appears to have three leaflets because of the presence of a raphe (*arrow*). **D:** PSAX in systole, "football"-shaped opening with fusion of right and left cusps. (*continued*)

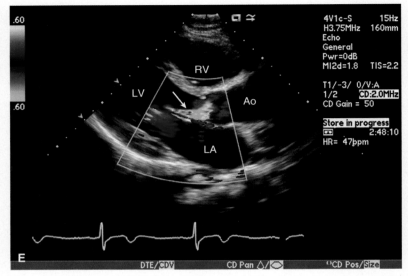

**Figure 9-2.** (*Continued*) (**E**) PLAX in diastole with color Doppler showing eccentric posteriorly directed AR (*arrow*).

○ **Aortic root dimension**
  - Measure the dimension of the *sinuses of Valsalva, sinotubular junction,* and *ascending aorta during systole (i.e., when the aortic valve is open)* (Fig. 9-3).
  - Particularly **important in Marfan's syndrome** (these patients develop a **"pear-shaped"** dilation of the aorta involving more of the sinuses and sinotubular junction than ascending aorta) **and BAV** (these patients can develop dilation of the aorta in the sinuses, sinotubular junction, or ascending aorta); aortic dilation predisposes to dissection and rupture.

○ **Left ventricular outflow tract dimension**
  - Cause for significant source of error in the measurement of AVA in patients with AS (error is squared in the continuity equation!).
  - Measure in the zoomed PLAX view during mid-systole (i.e., aortic leaflets are open).
  - Measure just proximal to the aortic valve and parallel to the aortic valve plane.
  - The LVOT dimension is often ~2.0 cm (usual range: 1.6 to 2.4 cm), but precise measurement is critical and **should be reported** to increase accuracy of serial comparison of calculated valve areas (i.e., the LVOT dimension should remain constant during serial evaluations).

○ **Aortic annulus dimension**
  - Measure from leaflet insertion to leaflet insertion.
  - This dimension is critical when considering transcatheter aortic valve replacement as it helps in the estimation of the size of the valve needed for implantation.

# Parasternal long-axis view

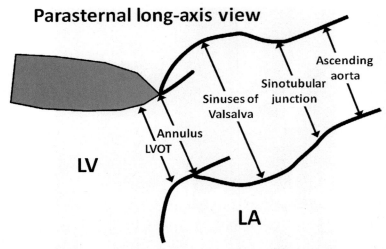

**Figure 9-3.** Left ventricular outflow and aortic root structures as a guide to location of measurements in a standard or high PLAX view.

○ **Left ventricular dimensions**
- Patients with AS can develop significant ventricular hypertrophy and eventually dilation. This can have important management implications.
○ **Left ventricular function**
- LVEF is an important parameter to follow in patients with AS; even in asymptomatic patients, an LVEF ≤50% is a Class 1 indication for surgery.
• **Doppler assessment**
○ **PW Doppler in the LVOT**
- In the apical three- or five-chamber view, place the sample volume in the LVOT just proximal to the aortic valve such that only the closing click is seen and there is no spectral broadening or "feathering" of the Doppler profile (Fig. 9-4).

> • **Key Point:** *Incorrect PW Doppler location can lead to velocity time integral (VTI) and velocity measurement errors reducing the accuracy of the reported valve area using the continuity equation. Occasionally, as a "reality check" a very bright inner envelope is seen on CW through the aortic valve that is representative of what the LVOT velocity and VTI should be (Fig. 9-5).*

○ **CW Doppler through the aortic valve**
- It is important to acquire the CW Doppler tracing from several locations (apex, suprasternal notch, and right parasternal) to ensure that the beam is parallel to the flow and the maximum jet velocity is obtained. The non-imaging probe (pedoff) should be used in each of these locations (Fig. 9-6).
○ **Mean and peak aortic valve gradients**
- Obtained when the CW Doppler signal is traced.

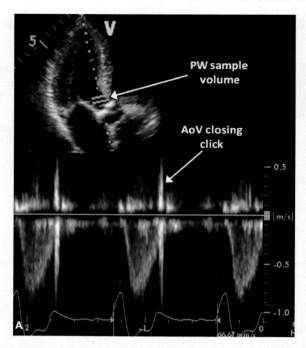

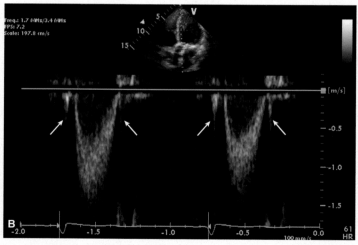

**Figure 9-4. A:** Correct positioning of the sample volume during PW Doppler acquisition in the LVOT so that only the closing click of the aortic valve is seen and there is little spectral broadening. **B:** Incorrect positioning of the sample volume too close to the aortic valve. Spectral Doppler shows both the opening and closing clicks of the aortic valve (*arrows*) and broadening of the Doppler jet, leading to overestimation of the VTI.

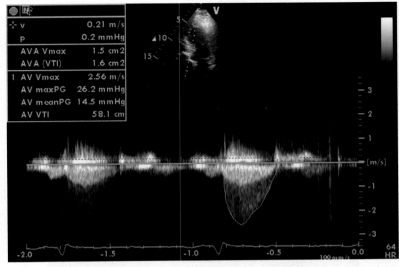

| v | 0.21 m/s |
| P | 0.2 mmHg |
| AVA Vmax | 1.5 cm2 |
| AVA (VTI) | 1.6 cm2 |
| AV Vmax | 2.56 m/s |
| AV maxPG | 26.2 mmHg |
| AV meanPG | 14.5 mmHg |
| AV VTI | 58.1 cm |

**Figure 9-5.** CW Doppler across the LVOT showing two envelopes: Lighter envelope that is traced represents flow velocities across the aortic valve, brighter inner envelope represents flow velocities across LVOT.

- Peak gradient is calculated using peak velocity in the modified Bernoulli equation: $\Delta P = 4v^2$.
- Mean gradient reflects the average gradient between the LV and aorta during systole; it is calculated by averaging the instantaneous gradients over the ejection period and requires tracing of the aortic Doppler envelope in order for machine calculation (Fig. 9-6).
- **Severe AS: Mean gradient >40 mmHg**

  - **Key Point:** *Be sure to trace the modal (bright and clearly defined) Doppler envelope when measuring gradients. Spectral broadening or "feathering" of the envelope line can be exacerbated by contrast or inappropriate Doppler settings leading to overestimation of gradients.*

○ **Aortic valve area**
  - Calculated based on the continuity equation, which holds that the volume of blood ejected through the LVOT equals the volume of blood that crosses the aortic valve: AVA × $VTI_{AoV}$ = (calculated surface area) $CSA_{LVOT}$ × $VTI_{LVOT}$ (Fig. 9-7).
  - Solving for AVA, yields: AVA = $CSA_{LVOT}$ × $VTI_{LVOT}/VTI_{AoV}$.
  - Should index to body surface area (BSA) if patient at extremes of body habitus.
  - **Severe AS: AVA <1 cm², AVA/BSA <0.6 cm²/m²**
○ **Dimensionless index**
  - Since inaccurate measurement of the LVOT diameter leads to wide variability of calculated AVA an index has been developed that does not rely on the diameter measurement.

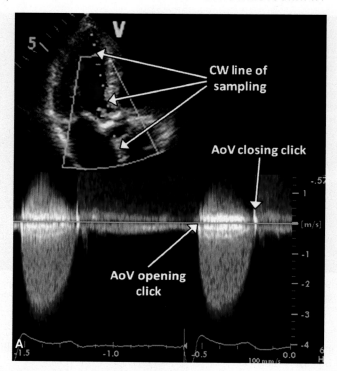

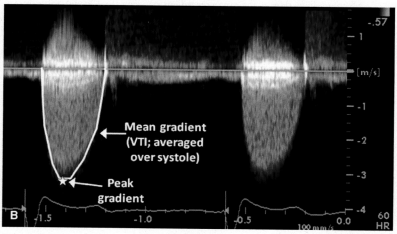

Figure 9-6. **A:** CW Doppler across the aortic valve allowing the highest velocity to be recorded. **B:** Measurement of mean and peak gradients from tracing the Doppler envelope.

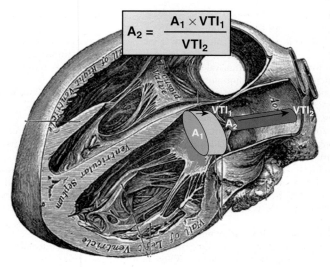

$$A_2 = \frac{A_1 \times VTI_1}{VTI_2}$$

**Figure 9-7.** Measurements used in the continuity equation to calculate AVA.

- This index takes the ratio of LVOT and AoV peak velocities or VTIs.
 - **Severe AS: LVOT/AoV VTI ratio <0.25, mild AS: LVOT/AoV VTI ratio >0.5.**
 ○ **Atrial fibrillation (and other irregular rhythms)**
 - Measure the VTI of the LVOT and AV from at least five successive beats and average the results for the determination of gradients and AVA.
• **Exercise testing**
 ○ When deciding the optimal timing of surgical intervention and the presence of symptoms is unclear, patients with severe AS may undergo an exercise stress test to assess functional capacity, symptoms, blood pressure response to exercise, and EKG changes.
• **Low-dose dobutamine echocardiography for low flow, low gradient reduced LVEF AS**
 ○ *Clinical problem:* In patients with significant LV dysfunction and reduced blood flow, the gradient generated across the aortic valve is often less than what is usually observed in severe AS (>40 mmHg). **Low flow, low gradient, low LVEF severe AS is usually defined by: AVA <1 cm²; LVEF <40%; and mean gradient <30 to 40 mmHg.** Pseudosevere AS is where the reduced opening of the AoV is not primarily related to stiffened leaflets (as in "true" severe AS) but the inability of the LV to generate high enough transvalvular blood flow to fully open the leaflets. Differentiating "true" severe AS from pseudosevere AS is crucial to determining patient suitability for aortic valve replacement.
 ○ *Why perform a dobutamine echocardiogram?* Dobutamine can enhance contractility and heart rate, both of which can increase transvalvular flow rate. This helps

determine: (1) Whether contractile reserve is present; and (2) whether there is true severe AS versus pseudosevere AS.

- ○ *Contractile reserve:* An increase in stroke volume ($CSA_{LVOT} \times VTI_{LVOT}$) by ≥20% with dobutamine; other measures include an improvement in wall motion, LVEF, or transvalvular flow rate. The absence of contractile reserve increases operative mortality.
- ○ *Severe versus pseudosevere AS:* True severe AS is defined by: <0.3 cm² increase in AVA and final AVA ≤1 cm² with dobutamine.

- **Low flow, low gradient *normal* LVEF AS**
  - ○ *Clinical problem:* Seen in patients with normal to increased left ventricular ejection fraction (LVEF) with significant LV concentric remodeling and **small cavity size** such that the total ventricular blood volume is markedly reduced. This reduced volume results in reduced transvalvular blood flow and transvalvular gradients despite the presence of significant AS and normal LVEF. If the calculated AVA is in the severe category these patients have a similarly poor prognosis as patients with severe AS and markedly elevated gradients.

- **Correlation with invasive measurements**
  - ○ A well-performed echocardiogram almost always provides adequate information for clinical management. When non-invasive testing is inconclusive or when there is a discrepancy between non-invasive tests and clinical findings regarding AS severity, invasive hemodynamics in the catheterization lab may be useful.
  - ○ When comparing echocardiography-derived and invasive measurements, it is important to remember:
    - Reliable invasive hemodynamics require the use of a dual-lumen pressure catheter to measure simultaneous pressures in the LV and aorta and not just an LV-to-aorta "pull back".
    - Invasive hemodynamics utilize the Gorlin formula for a calculation of AVA, which is flow dependent and, itself, prone to various sources of error.
    - The popular peak-to-peak gradient measured invasively is a non-physiologic value and is not the same as the peak instantaneous gradient measured by echocardiography (which will always be higher) (see Chapter 13, Fig. 13-6). Peak *instantaneous* gradients are comparable between both modalities.
    - Lower gradients measured invasively may result from **pressure recovery**, a phenomenon in which kinetic energy of the blood stream distal to the stenosis is recovered as pressure. As Doppler estimates the maximum pressure difference immediately distal to the valve, the pressure difference will be higher than when measured slightly downstream invasively when the pressure has been fully recovered. This is important in patients with small aortic roots (<3 cm).
    - **The mean transvalvular gradient is the best comparative measure between invasive and non-invasive techniques.**

- **Natural history**
  - • AS is a progressive disease typically characterized by an asymptomatic phase until the valve area is generally <1 cm². In the absence of symptoms, patients with AS have an overall good prognosis with a risk of sudden death estimated to be <1% per year.

- Predictors of decreased event-free survival (free of aortic valve replacement (AVR) or death) include: Higher peak aortic jet velocity, increased valve calcification, and coexistent CAD. Once patients experience symptoms, their average survival is 2 to 3 years with a high risk of sudden death.

## AORTIC REGURGITATION

- **Pathophysiology**
  - **Acute AR**

Sudden large regurgitant volume imposed on LV of
normal (or small) size with normal (or decreased) compliance
↓
Rapid ↑LVEDP and ↑LAP
LV attempts to maintain CO with ↑HR and ↑contractility
↓
Attempts to maintain forward SV/CO may be inadequate

| Pulmonary edema (↑LVEDP and ↑LAP) | Cardiogenic shock (↓forward SV/CO) ↑myocardial O₂ demand | Myocardial ischemia (↓coronary perfusion pressure) |

LV, left ventricle; LVEDP, left ventricular end-diastolic pressure; LAP, left atrial pressure; CO, cardiac output; HR, heart rate; SV, stroke volume.

  - **Chronic AR**

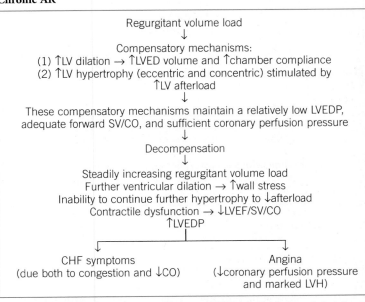

Regurgitant volume load
↓
Compensatory mechanisms:
(1) ↑LV dilation → ↑LVED volume and ↑chamber compliance
(2) ↑LV hypertrophy (eccentric and concentric) stimulated by ↑LV afterload
↓
These compensatory mechanisms maintain a relatively low LVEDP,
adequate forward SV/CO, and sufficient coronary perfusion pressure
↓
Decompensation
↓
Steadily increasing regurgitant volume load
Further ventricular dilation → ↑wall stress
Inability to continue further hypertrophy to ↓afterload
Contractile dysfunction → ↓LVEF/SV/CO
↑LVEDP

| CHF symptoms (due both to congestion and ↓CO) | Angina (↓coronary perfusion pressure and marked LVH) |

LV, left ventricle; LVED, left ventricular end diastolic; LVEDP, left ventricular end-diastolic pressure; EF, ejection fraction; SV, stroke volume; CO, cardiac output; CHF, congestive heart failure.

- **Etiology**

Aortic regurgitation (AR) results from pathology affecting the aortic valve and/or the supporting aortic root. AR usually develops insidiously, but may be acute.

| | |
|---|---|
| **More common** | • BAV<br>• Rheumatic disease<br>• Calcific degeneration<br>• Infective endocarditis<br>• Idiopathic aortic dilation<br>• Myxomatous degeneration<br>• Systemic hypertension<br>• Dissection of the ascending aorta<br>• Marfan's syndrome |
| **Less common** | • Traumatic injury<br>• Collagen vascular disease (ankylosing spondylitis, rheumatoid arthritis, Reiter's syndrome, giant cell arteritis, Whipple's disease)<br>• Syphilitic aortitis<br>• Osteogenesis imperfect<br>• Ehlers–Danlos syndrome<br>• Subaortic membrane<br>• Supra-cristal VSD leading to prolapse of an aortic cusp<br>• Anorectic drugs |
| **Acute** | • Infective endocarditis<br>• Dissection of the ascending aorta<br>• Trauma |

- **Echocardiographic assessment of AR**
  - **2D assessment**
    - **Leaflets**
      - Motion of the valve—is there prolapse of one of the leaflets?
      - Leaflet number—for example, eccentric AR with BAV?
      - Is there anything "extra" attached to the leaflets—for example, vegetation?
      - Calcification?
    - **Aortic root dimensions and morphology**
      - Is the support structure of the valve intact? Is there a suggestion of dissection? Is the root dilated?

      > • **Key Point:** *For complete aortic root measurement often moving the probe one intercostal space higher or tilting medially will offer better visualization and acoustic definition.*

    - **Left ventricular dimensions**
      - In chronic AR the ventricle will dilate; the left ventricular end-systolic diameter (LVESD) and left ventricular end-diastolic diameter (LVEDD) are important to follow in these patients → once the **LVESD reaches 5.0 cm** or the LVEDD reaches 7.0 cm, surgery should be considered even in asymptomatic patients.

- In chronic AR, the ventricle develops **eccentric hypertrophy** (LV mass is increased, wall thickness increases, and the chamber dilates) (see Chapter 4, Table 4-4).
○ **Left ventricular function**
   - In chronic AR, the LVEF can remain relatively normal for a long period of time; however, surgery should be performed when the **LVEF is ≤50%** even in asymptomatic patients.
   - **If the ventricle is normal size and hyperdynamic and the AR appears severe, the onset of the regurgitation is likely acute or subacute.**
• **Doppler assessment:** A number of variables can affect the Doppler assessment of AR including: Volume status, filling pressures, eccentricity of the jet, coexisting regurgitant or stenotic valve lesions, and blood pressure. It is critical to *integrate all the information* obtained from the echocardiogram to determine the severity of regurgitation.
○ **Qualitative**
   - **Color Doppler jet width**
     ▪ **Width of the color jet versus width of the LVOT**
     ▪ Less accurate with highly eccentric jets (tends to underestimate severity).
     ▪ Measure in the parasternal long- or short-axis view (zoomed) or in the 120-degree long-axis view in TEE. (*Note:* Due to reduced lateral beam resolution the jet will always seem broader in the apical views and therefore may be overestimated.)
     ▪ **<25% = mild AR; ≥65% = severe AR**
     ▪ **The length of the AR jet should not be used to assess AR severity** as it depends more on the driving pressure across the regurgitant orifice rather than the size of the orifice.
   - **Doppler vena contracta width**
     ▪ **Narrowest diameter of the regurgitant flow stream** and reflects the diameter of the regurgitant orifice. It is relatively load and flow rate independent.
     ▪ For accurate measurement you should be able to **identify all three components of the regurgitant jet** (i.e., proximal flow convergence, vena contracta, broadening in the LVOT). This avoids erroneously measuring the jet as it rapidly expands in the LVOT as the vena contracta.
     ▪ Avoid overestimation of vena contracta by measuring **only the high velocity color width** and not lower velocity blood that is drawn to the regurgitant jet stream.
     ▪ Measure in the parasternal long- or short-axis view (zoomed) or in the 120-degree long-axis view in TEE.
     ▪ **Vena contracta <0.3 cm = mild AR; vena contracta >0.6 cm = severe AR** (Fig. 9-8).
   - **Pressure half time (PHT)**
     ▪ **Time it takes for the pressure difference between the aorta and LV to decrease by one-half during diastole.**
     ▪ Easy to measure using CW Doppler in the three- or five-chamber views.
     ▪ The intensity/density of the signal of the regurgitant Doppler profile is also a qualitative sign of the amount of AR.
     ▪ Can be influenced by numerous factors including LV compliance, LV filling pressure, presence of significant MR, and the chronicity of AR.

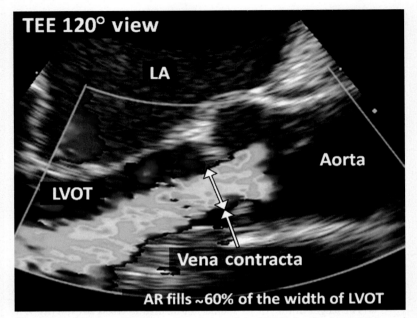

**Figure 9-8.** TEE long-axis mid-esophageal view of the LVOT showing image AR jet and measurement of the vena contracta.

- **PHT <200 ms = severe AR, PHT >500 ms = mild AR** (Fig. 9-9).
- Diastolic flow reversal in aorta
  - Aortic flow reversal can be assessed with PW Doppler in the proximal descending thoracic aorta (suprasternal view) or in the abdominal aorta (in the subcostal view).
  - **Holodiastolic flow reversal suggests at least moderate AR** with the greatest specificity being the presence of holodiastolic flow reversal in the abdominal aorta (Fig. 9-10).
  - Severe AR is suggested when the VTI of flow reversal approaches the VTI of forward flow in the aorta.

  > • Key Point: *Early, brief diastolic flow reversal may be seen, especially in young patients with compliant aortas and is NORMAL. It is important to distinguish this flow from HOLOdiastolic flow reversal, which is always ABNORMAL.*

- ○ **Quantitative:** Unlike mitral regurgitation, methods to quantify AR volume, while feasible, are not as frequently done. The severity of AR can often be determined by a combination of qualitative methods and the 2D assessment as above.
  - Proximal isovelocity surface area (PISA)
    - Regurgitant flow accelerates in layers or "surfaces" as it approaches the regurgitant orifice. Using color Doppler with a lowered aliasing velocity, the red–blue interface can be identified. The distance between the red–blue interface and the regurgitant orifice is the PISA radius. The PISA is the surface

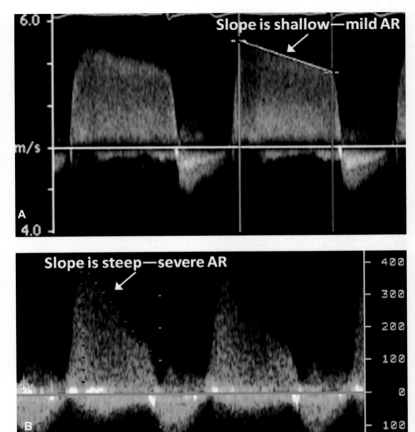

Figure 9-9. Measurement of PHT of AR jet suggesting (A) mild or (B) severe regurgitation.

area of blood moving back from the aorta toward the closed aortic valve at the given aliasing velocity.

- $PISA = 2\pi \times (PISA \text{ radius})^2$.
- Although difficult to measure this should be performed on a "zoomed" apical five or apical long-axis view.
- **Regurgitant volume (RegurgV)**
  - The volume of blood that regurgitates across the valve per beat
  - Calculated by three methods:
    □ Difference between transaortic and transmitral volume flow measured by PW Doppler.
      • Transaortic volume is $SV_{total}$ (forward and regurgitant volumes) and transmitral volume is $SV_{forward}$ (forward volume only).
      • $SV_{total} = CSA_{LVOT} \times VTI_{LVOT}$.
      • $SV_{forward} = CSA_{mitral\ annulus} \times VTI_{mitral\ annulus}$.

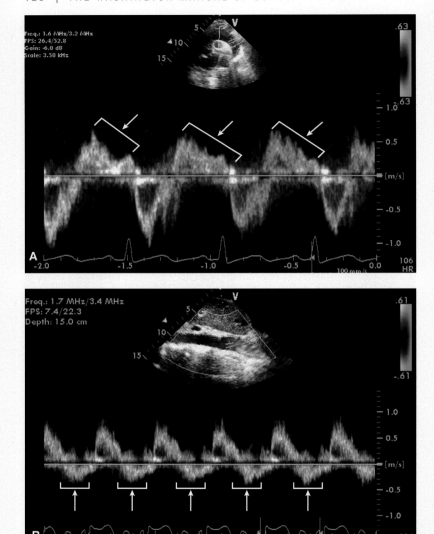

**Figure 9-10.** PW Doppler in the **(A)** proximal descending thoracic aorta and **(B)** abdominal aorta showing holodiastolic flow reversal (*arrows*) with similar VTI to forward flow suggestive of severe AR.

*Note: Use PW Doppler at the level of the mitral annulus.*
- $RegurgV = SV_{total} - SV_{forward}$.
- Not valid when significant MR present.

□ Another method for calculating $SV_{total}$ uses 2D measurement of LV volumes.
  - $SV_{total} = LVEDV - LVESV$ (by Simpson's method).
  - $RegurgV = SV_{total} - SV_{forward}$.
  - $RegurgV = 2D$ LV stroke volume $-$ $Volume_{transmitral}$

□ PISA
  - $RegurgV = EROA \times VTI_{AR\ jet}$.

■ **RegurgV <30 mL/beat = mild AR, RegurgV ≥60 mL/beat = severe AR.**
- **Regurgitant fraction (RegurgF)**
  ■ The ratio of the regurgitant flow to antegrade flow across the valve.
  ■ $RegurgF = RegurgV/SV_{total}$ (where $SV_{total} = CSA_{LVOT} \times VTI_{LVOT}$).
  ■ **RegurgF <30% = mild AR, RegurgF ≥50% = severe AR.**
- **Effective regurgitant orifice area (EROA):** The area of the regurgitant orifice.
  ■ $EROA = PISA \times$ aliasing velocity/peak AR velocity.
    OR
  ■ $EROA = RegurgV/VTI_{AR\ jet}$.
  ■ **EROA <0.1 cm² = mild AR, EROA ≥0.3 cm² = severe AR.**
- **TEE**
  ○ Can complement TTE in the assessment of AR.
  ○ Provides better visualization of the valve morphology and aortic root dimension; for example, endocarditis, aortic dissection.
- **Natural history**
See Table 9-4.

| **TABLE 9-4** | **Natural History of Aortic Regurgitation** |
|---|---|
| **Asymptomatic patients with normal LV systolic function** | |
| Progression to symptoms and/or LV dysfunction | <6% per year |
| Progression to asymptomatic LV dysfunction | <3.5% per year |
| Sudden death | <0.2% per year |
| **Asymptomatic patients with LV dysfunction** | |
| Progression to cardiac symptoms | >25% per year |
| **Symptomatic patients** | |
| Mortality rate | >10% per year |

LV, left ventricle.

From Bonow RO, Carabello BA, Chatterjee K, et al. ACC/AHA 2006 guidelines for the management of patients with valvular heart disease. *JACC.* 2006;48(3):e1–e148, with permission from Elsevier.

# Mitral Valve Disease

Brian R. Lindman and Suzanne V. Arnold

## HIGH-YIELD CONCEPTS

- Discrepancy between the mitral valve area (MVA) and mean gradient in MS may be related to cardiac output or heart rate
- *Wilkins score:* Carefully review leaflet mobility, thickening, and calcification and subvalvular thickening to predict efficacy of balloon valvuloplasty
- *Eccentric regurgitant jet:* Be suspicious that it might be severe
- *Grading regurgitation severity:* Do not rely on one measurement alone

## KEY VIEWS

- *Parasternal long axis*—initial screening for mitral stenosis (MS) and mitral regurgitation (MR) severity; evaluation of subvalvular apparatus
- *Parasternal short axis*—planimetry of MVA
- *Apical views*—quantitative assessment MS and MR: Mean gradient, proximal isovelocity surface area (PISA) and volumetric assessments, LA and LV size and function
- *TEE*—higher resolution views for MR etiology and severity (e.g., PISA, pulmonary vein reversal) and for Wilkins score; important for planning interventions

## SEVERITY OF MITRAL STENOSIS

See Table 10-1.

| TABLE 10-1 | Criteria for Determining Severity of Mitral Valve Stenosis | | |
| --- | --- | --- | --- |
| | **Mild** | **Moderate** | **Severe** |
| MVA (cm$^2$) | >1.5 | 1.0–1.5 | <1.0 |
| Mean gradient (mmHg) | <5 | 5–10 | >10 |
| PASP (mmHg) | >30 | 30–50 | >50 |

MVA, mitral valve area; PASP, pulmonary artery systolic pressure.

Adapted from Baumgartner H, Hung J, Bermejo J, et al. Echocardiographic assessment of valve stenosis: EAE/ASE recommendations for clinical practice. *J Am Soc Echocardiogr.* 2009;22(1):1–23, with permission from Elsevier.

## SEVERITY OF MITRAL REGURGITATION

See Table 10-2.

| TABLE 10-2 | Criteria for Determining Severity of Mitral Valve Regurgitation | | |
|---|---|---|---|
| | **Mild** | **Moderate** | **Severe** |
| **Specific signs of severity** | • Small central jet <4 cm² or <20% of LA area[a] <br> • Vena contracta width <0.3 cm <br> • No or minimal flow convergence[b] | Signs of MR > mild present, but no criteria for severe MR | • Vena contracta width ≥0.7 cm *with* large central MR jet (area >40% of LA) or *with* a wall-impinging jet of any size, swirling in LA[a] <br> • Large flow convergence[b] <br> • Systolic reversal in pulmonary veins <br> • Prominent flail MV leaflet or ruptured papillary muscle |
| **Supportive signs** | • Systolic dominant flow in pulmonary veins <br> • A-wave dominant mitral inflow[c] <br> • Soft density, parabolic CW Doppler MR signal <br> • Normal LV size[d] | Intermediate signs/ findings | • Dense, triangular CW Doppler MR jet <br> • E-wave dominant mitral inflow (E >1.2 m/s)[c] Enlarged LV and LA size[e], (particularly when normal LV function is present). |
| **Quantitative parameters[f]** | | | |
| R Vol (mL/beat) | <30 | 30–44 | 45–59    ≥60 |
| RF (%) | <30 | 30–39 | 40–49    ≥50 |
| EROA (cm²) | <0.20 | 0.20–0.29 | 0.30–0.39    ≥0.40 |

CW, continuous wave; EROA, effective regurgitant orifice area; LA, left atrium; LV, left ventricle; MV, mitral valve; MR, mitral regurgitation; R Vol, regurgitant volume; RF, regurgitant fraction.

[a]At a Nyquist limit of 50 to 60 cm/s.

[b]Minimal and large flow convergence defined as a flow convergence radius <0.4 cm and ≥0.9 cm for central jets, respectively, with a baseline shift at a Nyquist of 40 cm/s; Cut-offs for eccentric jets are higher, and should be angle corrected (see text).

[c]Usually above 50 years of age or in conditions of impaired relaxation, in the absence of mitral stenosis or other causes of elevated LA pressure.

[d]LV size applies only to chronic lesions. Normal 2D measurements: LV minor axis ≤2.8 cm/m², LV end-diastolic volume ≤82 mL/m², maximal LA antero-posterior diameter ≤2.8 cm/m², maximal LA volume ≤36 mL/m² (2;33;35).

[e]In the absence of other etiologies of LV and LA dilatation and acute MR.

[f]Quantitative parameters can help subclassify the moderate regurgitation group into mild-to-moderate and moderate-to-severe as shown.

Adapted from Zoghbi WA, Enriquez-Sarano M, Foster E, et al. Recommendations for evaluation of the severity of native valvular regurgitation with two-dimensional and Doppler echocardiography. *J Am Soc Echocardiogr.* 2003;16(7):777–802, with permission from Elsevier.

## ANATOMY

- **Leaflets**
  - Anterior and posterior leaflets each have three scallops (Fig. 10-1).
- **Annulus**
  - The junction between atrium and ventricle and the place where the mitral leaflets insert.
  - There is an anterior and posterior portion of the annulus corresponding to the respective leaflets. The anterior portion is attached to the right and left fibrous trigones and is structurally more supported.
  - The annulus may dilate leading to functional regurgitation or calcify leading to stenosis.
- **Subvalvular Apparatus**
  - Papillary muscles: Anterior–lateral and posterior–medial; the anterior–lateral papillary muscle usually receives dual blood supply (LAD and LCX), whereas the posterior–medial papillary muscle usually has single blood supply (either LCX or RCA).
  - Chordae tendinae: Primary, secondary, and tertiary chords connect the papillary muscles to **both** valve leaflets; these can elongate, shorten, rupture, calcify, or fuse.
- **Ventricle**
  - The ventricular size and shape impact the function of the mitral valve. As the ventricle dilates and becomes more spherical, the papillary muscles become apically displaced and can restrict the closure of the mitral leaflets, leading to MR.

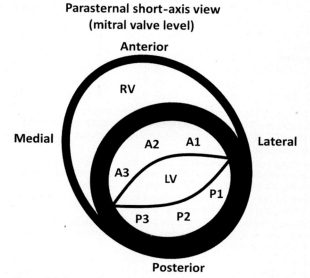

**Parasternal short-axis view (mitral valve level)**

Anterior

RV

Medial — Lateral

A2  A1

A3  LV  P1

P3  P2

Posterior

Figure 10-1. Cartoon of parasternal short axis at the mitral valve level showing the different scallops numbered in ascending order from lateral to medial.

- **Left Atrium**
  - If the left atrium dilates, this can lead to annular dilation and affect the closure of the mitral leaflets, leading to MR.

  > - **Key Point:** *Unlike the tricuspid and pulmonic valve, which is separated by the RV infundibulum the mitral and aortic valve, are in direct continuity, separated only by a fibrous connection. This has ramifications for pathology such as endocarditis, which can therefore spread between both valves and cause annular and aortic root abscess.*

## MITRAL STENOSIS

- **Pathophysiology**
  See Figure 10-2.
- **Etiology**

| | |
|---|---|
| **Rheumatic (most common)** | • 2/3 are female<br>• May be associated with MR<br>• Stenotic orifice often shaped like a "fish mouth" (PSAX) (Fig. 10-3) with doming of anterior leaflet (PLAX and apical views) (Fig. 10-4) and marked reduction in posterior leaflet motion<br>• Rheumatic fever can cause fibrosis, thickening, and calcification leading to fusion of the commissures, cusps, and/or chordae.<br>• As opposed to calcific MS this process starts in the subvalvular apparatus and extends to the leaflets with increasingly severe disease. |
| **Other causes (less common)** | • Congenital<br>• Mitral annular calcification (i.e., calcific MS)—process starts from annulus and extends to the leaflets. Significant calcification is required to impact the larger area of the mitral annulus compared to rheumatic MS which affects the leaflet tips<br>• Chest radiation<br>• MV prosthesis dysfunction<br>• Mucopolysaccharidoses<br>• Malignant carcinoid<br>• Systemic lupus erythematosus (SLE)<br>• Rheumatoid arthritis<br>• Iatrogenic due to surgery for MR: Oversewn mitral annuloplasty ring, MV clip/Alfieri stitch<br>• "Functional MS" due to restriction of left atrial outflow (MV leaflets are normal):<br>  – Tumor (typically atrial myxoma)<br>  – LA thrombus<br>  – Endocarditis with large vegetation<br>  – Cor triatriatum (congenital LA membrane) |

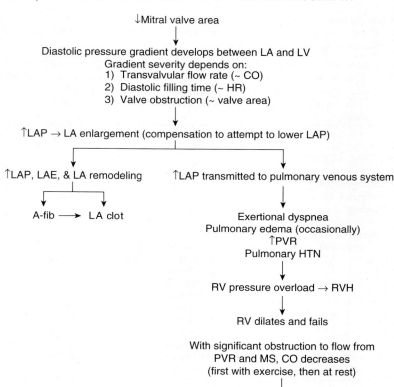

↓Mitral valve area

↓

Diastolic pressure gradient develops between LA and LV
Gradient severity depends on:
1) Transvalvular flow rate (~ CO)
2) Diastolic filling time (~ HR)
3) Valve obstruction (~ valve area)

↓

↑LAP → LA enlargement (compensation to attempt to lower LAP)

↑LAP, LAE, & LA remodeling          ↑LAP transmitted to pulmonary venous system

↓                                    ↓

A-fib ⟶ LA clot                     Exertional dyspnea
                                     Pulmonary edema (occasionally)
                                     ↑PVR
                                     Pulmonary HTN

                                     ↓

                                     RV pressure overload → RVH

                                     ↓

                                     RV dilates and fails

                                     With significant obstruction to flow from
                                     PVR and MS, CO decreases
                                     (first with exercise, then at rest)

                                     ↓

                                     Fatigue, dyspnea, ↓functional capacity

LA, left atrium; LV, left ventricle; CO, cardiac output; HR, heart rate; LAP, left atrial pressure; LAE, left atrial enlargement; PVR, pulmonary vascular resistance; RV, right ventricle; RVH, right ventricular hypertrophy; CO, cardiac output.

**Figure 10-2.** The pathophysiology of mitral stenosis and associated echocardiographic features.

- **Echocardiographic assessment of MS**
- **2D assessment**
  - **Leaflets**
    - ○ Motion/mobility of the valve
    - ○ Thickening
    - ○ Calcification
  - **Subvalvular apparatus**
    - ○ Chordal fusion, shortening, fibrosis, and calcification
  - **Mitral valve area planimetry**
    - ○ The mitral valve orifice is traced in the parasternal short-axis view usually during mid-diastole.

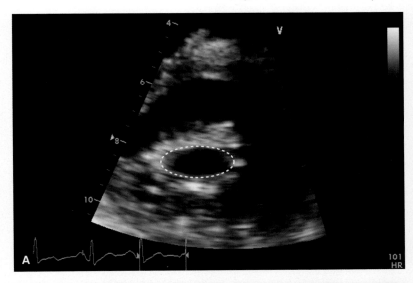

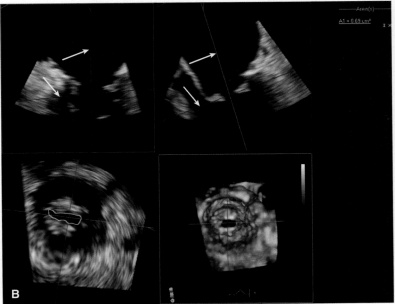

**Figure 10-3. A:** A 2D PSAX view at the MV leaflet tips with planimetry of the orifice in mid-diastole. **B:** 3D PSAX view for planimetry of a mitral valve that is severely stenotic. Note the ability to easily determine the correct position of the orifice in the 3D example by manipulation of the planes in the biplanar TEE images (*arrows*).

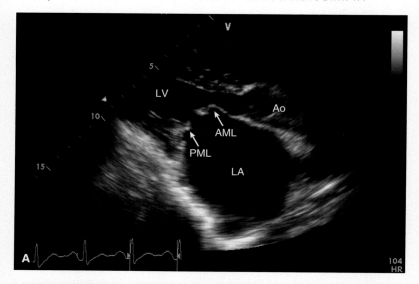

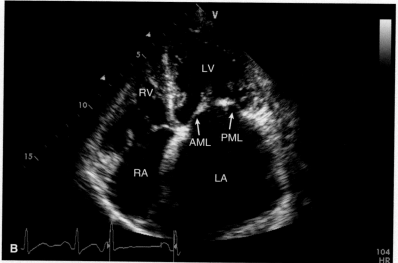

**Figure 10-4.** (A) Parasternal long-axis and (B) apical four-chamber views showing doming of the anterior mitral leaflet and a thickened and fixed posterior mitral leaflet consistent with rheumatic mitral valve disease (*arrows*).

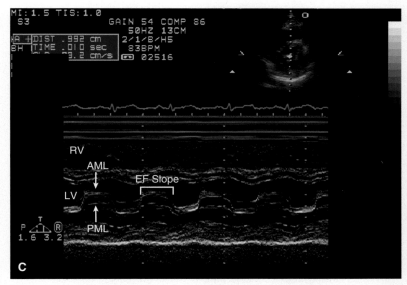

**Figure 10-4.** (*Continued*) (**C**) M-mode shows the classic features of thickened mitral valve leaflets, "tracking" of the posterior leaflet and reduced E-F slope.

- o This can be an accurate way to assess the severity of MS that is independent of flow, chamber compliance, and other valve lesions; however, it is also prone to error. While in the parasternal short-axis view, scanning should be done from apex to base to ensure that planimetry is being done at the leaflet tips. Sometime, reviewing the anatomy from the parasternal long-axis view can help identify the right plane in the short-axis view. This is a measurement where 3D imaging is particularly helpful in enhancing accuracy (Fig. 10-3).
- **Left atrial dimension**
  - Significant MS can lead to substantial dilation of the LA, predisposing the patient to atrial arrhythmias and thrombus formation.
  - **Wilkins score is graded as detailed in Table 10-3.**
- **Doppler**
  - **MVA**
    - o **Pressure half-time (PHT) method**
      - PHT is the time it takes for the pressure across the mitral valve to decrease by one-half its original maximal value; it is measured by tracing the deceleration slope of the E wave on the CW Doppler profile through the mitral valve.

---

- **Key Point:** *If the Doppler profile contains a brief steep slope and then longer less steep slope, measure the latter. The so called "ski slope" beginning is not indicative of the true gradient between LA and LV during filling.*

---

      - MVA = 220/PHT
      - PHT should not be used to estimate MVA in the following circumstances: Immediately post-valvuloplasty (first 72 hours), if MV is prosthetic, in the presence of an ASD, if severe AR is present or when LV filling pressures are very high (Fig. 10-5).

| TABLE 10-3 | Wilkins Score Grading | | |
|---|---|---|---|

| Grade | Mobility | Thickening | Calcification | Subvalvular thickening |
|---|---|---|---|---|
| 1 | Highly mobile valve with only leaflet tips restricted | Leaflets near normal in thickness (4–5 mm) | A single area of increased echo brightness | Minimal thickening just below the mitral leaflets |
| 2 | Leaflet mid and base portions have normal mobility | Midleaflets normal, considerable thickening of margins (5–8 mm) | Scattered areas of brightness confined to leaflet margins | Thickening of chordal structures extending to one-third of the chordal length |
| 3 | Valve continues to move forward in diastole mainly from the base | Thickening extending through the entire leaflet (5–8 mm) | Brightness extending into the mid-portions of the leaflets | Thickening extended to distal third of the chords |
| 4 | No or minimal forward movement of the leaflets in diastole | Considerable thickening of all leaflet tissue (>8–10 mm) | Extensive brightness throughout much of the leaflet tissue | Extensive thickening and shortening of all chordal structures extending down to the papillary muscles |

Adapted from Baumgartner H, Hung J, Bermejo J, et al. Echocardiographic assessment of valve stenosis: EAE/ASE recommendations for clinical practice. *J Am Soc Echocardiogr.* 2009;22(1):1–23, with permission from Elsevier.

○ **Continuity equation method**
  - This is analogous to measuring AVA utilizing measurements of the LVOT and AoV.
  - MVA = $\pi \times (D_{LVOT}/2)^2 \times (VTI_{LVOT}/VTI_{mitral})$ where $D_{LVOT}$ is the LVOT diameter (in cm), $VTI_{LVOT}$ is measured from the PW Doppler in the LVOT, and $VTI_{mitral}$ is measured from the CW Doppler through the MV.
  - Not accurate in the setting of atrial fibrillation or ≥ moderate MR or AR.
○ **PISA method**
  - Zoom view of mitral with baseline of the Nyquist limit moved in the direction of mitral inflow to allow earlier aliasing of color and a larger flow convergence radius (r) to be measured.
  - MVA = $(\pi r^2 \times V_{aliasing}/V_{peak\ mitral\ E}) \times \alpha/180°$

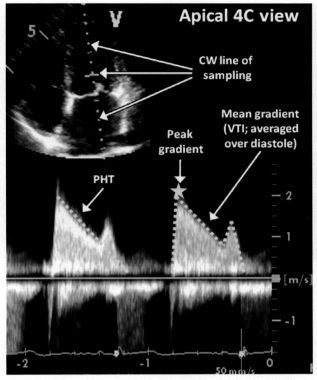

**Figure 10-5.** Continuous-wave Doppler of mitral inflow with pressure half time measured.

- Limited use because of errors in accurately measuring flow convergence radius (r) and opening angle of the mitral leaflets ($\alpha$).

- **Mean and peak mitral valve gradients**
  - The CW Doppler signal is obtained through the mitral valve in the apical window; this Doppler profile is traced for calculation of the gradient.
  - Peak gradient is calculated using peak velocity in the modified Bernoulli equation: $\Delta P = 4 \times v^2$.
  - Mean gradient reflects the average gradient between LA and LV during diastole; it is calculated by averaging the instantaneous gradients (tracing the CW Doppler MV envelope).

- **Mean gradient is more useful clinically**; however, it is important to realize that it is influenced by heart rate, diastolic filling time, cardiac output, and associated MR (Fig. 10-6).

- **Key Point:** *In reporting mitral valve gradients, the heart rate should always be included to allow comparison between serial studies and alert the referring physician to the influence that this may have on the diastolic filling period.*

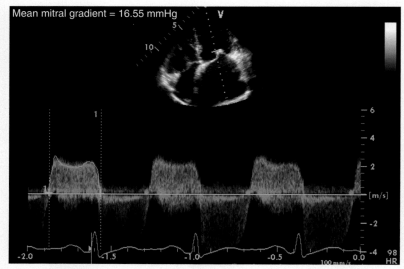

**Figure 10-6.** Continuous-wave Doppler of mitral inflow traced to measure the mean mitral gradient.

- **Pulmonary artery pressure**
  - The estimated pulmonary artery systolic pressure (PASP) and mean pulmonary artery pressure should be measured (see Chapter 5).
- **Atrial fibrillation (and other irregular rhythms)**
  - Average results over several beats (preferably five) when measuring PHT and mitral gradients.
- **TEE**
  - Provides a better look at the mitral valve and subvalvular anatomy to assess candidacy for percutaneous balloon valvuloplasty.
  - Assesses degree of associated MR.
  - Assesses for LA or LAA thrombus.
  - Usually less accurate than TTE in measurement of mitral valve gradients because of difficulty in ensuring Doppler interrogation is parallel to flow.

---

- **Key Point:** *Percutaneous balloon valvuloplasty is contraindicated if moderate to severe MR or left atrial thrombus is present.*

---

- **Exercise testing**
  - Can be very helpful to determine functional capacity and the hemodynamic impact of the stenotic mitral valve in the setting of exertion.
  - Measurement of **mean mitral valve gradient** and **pulmonary artery pressure** are the most important part of the exercise echocardiogram for patients with MS.

- **Correlation with invasive catheterization measurements**
  - Can be helpful in assessing the severity of MS when the clinical and echocardiographic assessments are discordant.
  - Can provide an invasive assessment of pulmonary artery pressures if they are unclear by echocardiography.
  - The mean mitral gradient is most accurately calculated with simultaneous pressure recordings in the LA (utilizing a trans-septal puncture) and the LV.
  - MVA is calculated using the Gorlin formula.
- **Natural history**
  - MS usually progresses slowly with a long latent period (several decades) between rheumatic fever and the development of orifice stenosis significant enough to cause symptoms (usually <2 to 2.5 $cm^2$ with exercise or <1.5 $cm^2$ at rest). Ten-year survival of untreated patients presenting with MS depends on the severity of symptoms at presentation: Asymptomatic or minimally symptomatic patients have an 80% 10-year survival, whereas those with significant limiting symptoms have a 0 to 15% 10-year survival. Once severe pulmonary HTN develops, mean survival is 3 years. The mortality of untreated patients is due mostly to progressive pulmonary and systemic congestion, systemic embolism, pulmonary embolism, and infection.

## MITRAL REGURGITATION

- **Pathophysiology**
  See Figure 10-7.
- **Etiology**

| | |
|---|---|
| **Degenerative/ mitral valve prolapse syndrome** | • Usually occurs as a primary condition (Barlow's disease or fibroelastic deficiency) but has also been associated with heritable connective tissue disorders (e.g., Marfan's syndrome, Ehlers–Danlos syndrome, osteogenesis imperfecta). <br> • Occurs in 1–2.5% of the population <br> • Two-third are female <br> • Posterior leaflet (P2 scallop) most commonly prolapses (Fig. 10-8) <br> • Most common reason for MV surgery <br> • Myxomatous proliferation and cartilage formation can occur in the leaflets, chordae tendineae, and/or annulus |
| **Dilated cardiomyopathy** | • MR is due to both annular dilatation from LV enlargement and papillary muscle displacement from LV enlargement and spherical remodeling to prevent adequate leaflet coaptation <br> • May occur in nonischemic or ischemic dilated cardiomyopathy (there are often multiple mechanistic reasons for MR in the setting of prior infarction) |

| Ischemic | • *Ischemic MR is mostly a misnomer as this is primarily postinfarction MR, not MR caused by active ischemia* (although MR can be solely due to or exacerbated by ischemia)<br>• MR is primarily attributable to LV dysfunction—not papillary muscle dysfunction<br>• Mechanism of MR usually involves one or both of the following:<br>  – Annular dilatation from LV enlargement<br>  – Local LV remodeling with papillary muscle displacement (both the dilatation of the LV and the akinesis/dyskinesis of the wall to which the papillary muscle is attached can apically displace leaflet coaptation causing "tenting" of the leaflets) (Fig. 10-9)<br>• Rarely, MR may develop acutely from papillary muscle rupture (usually the posteromedial papillary muscle due to a single blood supply) |
|---|---|
| Rheumatic | • May be pure MR or combined MR/MS<br>• Caused by thickening and/or calcification of the leaflets and chordae |
| Infective endocarditis | • Usually caused by destruction of the leaflet tissue (i.e., perforation) |
| Other causes | • Congenital (e.g., cleft, parachute, or fenestrated MV)<br>• Infiltrative diseases (e.g., amyloid)<br>• SLE (i.e., Libman–Sacks lesion)<br>• Hypertrophic cardiomyopathy with LV outflow obstruction<br>• Mitral annular calcification<br>• Perivalvular MV prosthetic valve leak<br>• Drug toxicity (e.g., phen-fen) |
| Acute causes | • Ruptured papillary muscle<br>• Ruptured chordae tendineae<br>• Infective endocarditis |

## MITRAL REGURGITATION

• **2D assessment**
  • **Etiology**
    ○ Determining the etiology of MR by 2D, has important management implications (e.g., prolapse, leaflet tenting, ventricular shape and function, wall motion abnormalities, and papillary muscle displacement)
  • **Leaflets**
    ○ Motion of the valve (e.g., prolapse—leaflet body bows >1 mm behind annular plane; tenting—leaflet coaptation occurs further into LV; flail—leaflet tip points back to LA) (Fig. 10-10)

**Part A• Acute mitral regurgitation**

Sudden large volume load imposed on LA and
LV of normal size and compliance

↓

Rapid ↑LVEDP, ↑LAP
↑LV preload (from volume load) facilitates LV attempt to maintain forward
SV/CO with ↑HR and ↑contractility via Frank–Starling
mechanisms and catecholamines

↓

Attempts to maintain forward SV/CO may be inadequate despite a
supra-normal LVEF because a larger proportion is ejected backwards due
to the lower resistance of the LA

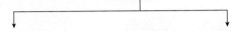

Pulmonary edema (↑LAP)              Hypotension (or shock) (↓forward SV/CO)


**Part B• Chronic mitral regurgitation**

Gradual volume load imposed on LA and LV

↓

↑LVEDP and ↑LAP

↓

Compensatory dilatation of the LA and LV to accommodate volume load at
lower pressures; this helps relieve pulmonary congestion
↑LV hypertrophy (eccentric) stimulated by LV dilatation (increased wall
stress – LaPlace's law)

↓

↑Preload, LV hypertrophy, and reduced or normal afterload
(low resistance LA provides unloading of LV) → large total
SV (supra-normal LVEF) and normal forward SV

↓

"MR begets more MR" (vicious cycle in which further
LV/annular dilatation ↔ ↑MR)

↓

Contractile dysfunction → ↓LVEF, ↑end-systolic volume → ↑LVEDP/volume, ↑LAP

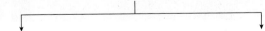

Pulmonary congestion & pHTN              Reduced forward SV/CO

LA, left atrium; LV, left ventricle; LVEDP, left ventricular end-diastolic pressure; LAP,
left atrial pressure; SV, stroke volume; CO, cardiac output; pHTN, pulmonary
hypertension.

Figure 10-7. **A:** Pathophysiology of acute MR and echocardiographic features.**B:** Pathophysiology of chronic MR and echocardiographic features.

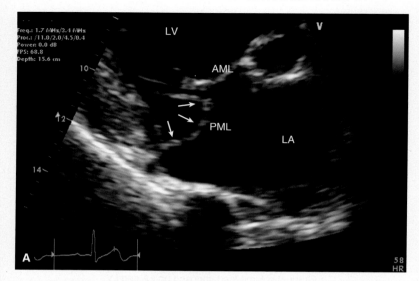

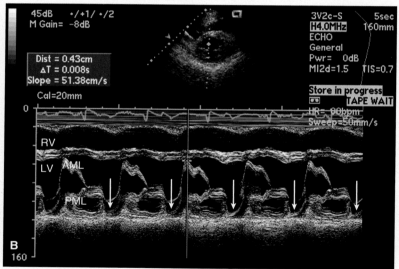

Figure 10-8. Posterior leaflet mitral valve prolapse (*arrows*) seen on (**A**) a zoomed 2D image in the parasternal long-axis view and (**B**) on M-mode echocardiography.

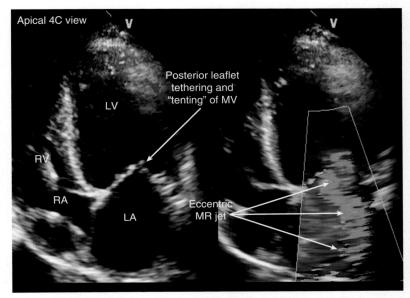

**Figure 10-9.** Tenting of the posterior mitral leaflet with apical displacement of leaflet coaptation resulting in eccentric posterior–lateral regurgitation.

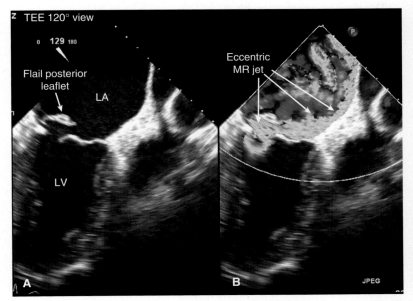

**Figure 10-10.** **(A)** Flail mitral valve with posterior leaflet pointing backward into LA. By definition this anatomic finding results in severe regurgitation as is seen in this case with color Doppler **(B)**.

○ Is there anything "extra" attached to the leaflets (e.g., vegetation) or a perforation?
○ Calcification

• **Subvalvular apparatus**
  ○ Papillary muscle displacement
  ○ Torn or elongated chordae tendineae

• **Mitral annulus**
  ○ Assess degree of dilation and/or calcification

• **Left atrial dimension**
  ○ Chronic severe MR will lead to enlargement of the left atrium; the LA dimensions and volume can elucidate the chronicity and degree of volume overload.

• **Left ventricular dimensions and function**
  ○ Measurement of the LV dimension at end-systole and end-diastole is important for assessing the ventricle's response to volume overload.
  ○ Chronic severe MR eventually leads to dilatation of the ventricle. An enlarged end-systolic dimension (≥4.0 cm) is an indication for surgery even in the absence of symptoms

• **Doppler**

• **Color Doppler jet area**
  ○ Color jet area depends on instrument settings, hemodynamics, jet eccentricity, orifice geometry, pulmonary venous counterflow, and left atrial compliance and must be interpreted with caution.
  ○ Measure in the apical four-chamber view and parasternal long-axis view; usually this is assessed qualitatively, but quantitative criteria are noted in Figure 10-1.

• **Doppler vena contracta width**
  ○ This is the narrowest diameter of the regurgitant flow stream and reflects the diameter of the regurgitant orifice. It is measured in the parasternal long-axis view in zoom mode and is the narrowest segment between the proximal flow convergence and the expansion of the regurgitant jet downstream. It is relatively load and flow rate independent (Fig. 10-11).

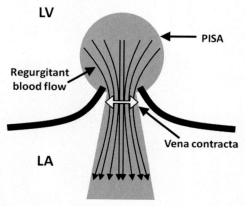

**Figure 10-11.** Cartoon showing flow convergence of mitral regurgitant blood and the narrowest portion of the jet as the blood enters the LA called the vena contracta.

- **Proximal isovelocity surface area (PISA)**
  - Regurgitant blood accelerates as "hemispheric layers" as it moves from the wider LV to the narrow mitral valve orifice.
  - When the velocity exceeds the nyquist limit it aliases; that is, changes from blue to red or red to blue depending on the direction of blood flow in relation to the probe.
  - Using the continuity principle the product of the surface area of the hemisphere as the blood aliases and the aliasing velocity must equal the product of the EROA and the velocity of blood moving through the orifice (peak MR velocity).
  - Surface area of a hemisphere = $2\pi r^2$
  - Effective regurgitant orifice area (EROA) = $2\pi r^2 \times$ aliasing velocity/peak MR velocity.

---

- **Key Point:** *To increase the PISA radius for accurate measurement the Nyquist limit baseline is moved in the direction of regurgitant blood flow so that the regurgitant blood aliases early. This direction therefore differs for TTE and TEE because of the different probe locations (Fig. 10-12).*

---

- **Regurgitant volume**
  - The volume of blood that regurgitates across the valve per beat or second
  - Calculated by three methods:
    - (1) Difference between transaortic and transmitral volume flow
    - $Volume_{transaortic} = CSA_{LVOT} \times VTI_{LVOT}$
    - $Volume_{transmitral} = CSA_{mitral\ annulus} \times VTI_{mitral\ annulus}$
    - *Use PW Doppler at the level of the mitral annulus*
    - Regurgitant volume (RegurgV) = $Volume_{transmitral} - Volume_{transaortic}$
    - Not valid in the setting of significant AR
    - (2) Difference between 2D LV stroke volume and forward stroke volume
    - 2D LV stroke volume = LVEDV − LVESV (modified Simpson's)
    - $SV_{forward} = CSA_{LVOT} \times VTI_{LVOT}$
    - RegurgV = 2D LV stroke volume − $SV_{forward}$
    - (3) PISA
    - EROA = $2\pi r^2 \times$ aliasing velocity/Peak MR velocity
    - RegurgV (mL) = EROA × $VTI_{MR\ jet}$
- **Regurgitant fraction**
  - The ratio of the regurgitant flow to antegrade flow across the valve
  - RF = RegurgV/$SV_{total}$ (where $SV_{total} = CSA_{mitral\ annulus} \times VTI_{mitral\ annulus}$)
- **EROA**
  - EROA = RegurgV/$VTI_{MR\ jet}$
- **Indirect measures**
  - In severe MR, the LA pressure is high; thus the E-wave in MV inflow should be high (>1.2 cm/s). E/A reversal pattern (impaired myocardial relaxation) on MV inflow virtually excludes severe MR.
  - The density (similar to inflow Doppler density) and shape (early peaking) of the MR jet on CW Doppler can be helpful.
    - The density/brightness of the CW Doppler envelope is proportional to the volume of blood. In severe MR, the MR jet is similar density to the MV inflow.
    - The MR jet velocity is determined by the pressure gradient between LV and LA. In severe (usually acute) MR, the LA pressure is very high, thus the pressure

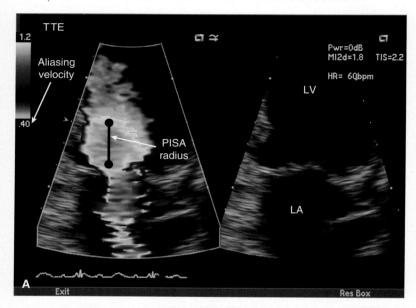

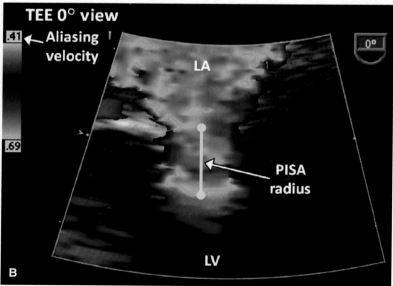

**Figure 10-12.** Measurement of PISA radius with (**A**) a zoomed TTE and (**B**) TEE view. Note that the Nyquist baseline is shifted based on the direction of the mitral valve regurgitation in relation to the different probe locations.

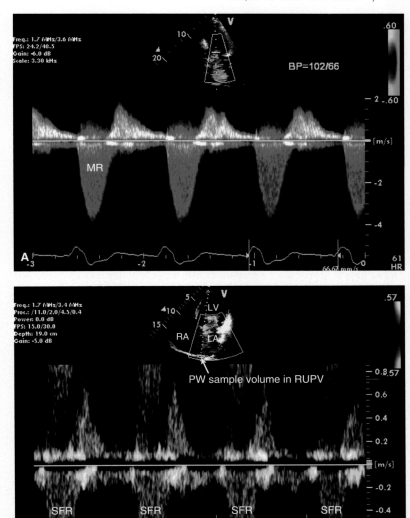

**Figure 10-13. (A)** Dense early peaking MR jet and **(B)** systolic flow reversal seen on PW Doppler sampling of the right upper pulmonary vein suggest severe MR.

difference between LV and LA will equilibrate quickly. This produces an MR jet with a sharp downslope in early systole (i.e., V-shaped) (Fig. 10-13A).
  ○ Systolic flow reversal may be seen in the pulmonary veins and suggests severe MR (Fig. 10-13B).
  ○ Pulmonary pressures are invariably elevated in chronic severe MR. When following a patient longitudinally with MR, an increase in PA pressures can be a marker that the MR has worsened.
- **TEE**
  - Can provide important complementary information (to TTE) in the assessment of patients with acute or chronic MR.
  - Valve leaflets are better visualized to clarify which scallops are prolapsed or flail.
  - Higher resolution images allow for more accurate assessment of PISA and vena contracta.
  - All the pulmonary veins can be interrogated for evidence of systolic flow reversal, a marker of severe MR.
  - Particularly helpful when assessing endocarditis, enabling an evaluation of the vegetation (size and mobility), leaflet damage (perforation), and extent of the infection (involvement of the fibrous continuum between the mitral and aortic valves with abscess or fistula formation).
- **Natural history**
  - The natural history and progression of MR depends on the etiology, associated LV dysfunction, and severity of MR at the time of diagnosis. Mitral valve prolapse with little or no MR most often has a benign prognosis and normal life expectancy; a minority of these patients will go on to develop severe MR (10% to15% of patients). The compensated asymptomatic phase of patients with severe MR with normal LV function is variable but may last several years. Factors independently associated with increased mortality after surgery includes: Preoperative EF <60% (expect hyperdynamic LV with severe MR), NYHA functional class III-IV symptoms, age, concomitant CAD, AF, and EROA >40 mm$^2$.

The natural history for ischemic MR and MR due to dilated cardiomyopathy (DCM) is generally worse than for degenerative MR because of the associated comorbidities in these patients. Ischemic MR is associated with increased mortality after MI, in chronic CHF, and after revascularization. Its impact on mortality increases with severity of regurgitation. Moreover, ischemic MR is an important predictor of future CHF. The presence of MR in the setting of DCM is common (up to 60% of patients) and associated with increased mortality. In both ischemic MR and MR due to DCM, because "MR begets MR" the ventricles of these patients dilate further and their CHF symptoms worsen as ventricular efficiency decreases.

# Pulmonic Valve

Anupama Rao

HIGH-YIELD FINDINGS

- Pulmonic stenosis (PS) is usually found in conjunction with **congenital heart disease**
- PS may occur at the valvular, subvalvular, or supravalvular levels
- Carcinoid disease is a common cause of **acquired** pulmonic valve disease and can cause both stenosis and regurgitation
- Severe pulmonic regurgitation (PR) is most often seen in the setting of pulmonary hypertension or in patients with repaired tetralogy of Fallot
- With severe PR, CW Doppler shows **rapid deceleration** of the PR jet. Presystolic forward flow can be seen with severe PR due to premature opening of PV due to high RVEDP

## KEY VIEWS

**TTE**
- PLAX and PSAX views tilted toward RV outflow tract (RVOT)
- Subcostal view

**TEE**
- High esophageal view at 0 to 20 degrees
- Mid esophageal level at 50 to 90 degrees (RV inflow/outflow view)
- Deep transgastric view 110 to 140 degrees

## ANATOMY

The pulmonic valve is a semi-lunar valve regulating flow between the right ventricle and the pulmonary artery. It consists of three leaflets projecting into the pulmonary artery, namely the anterior, right, and left cusps. The leaflets are attached at their base to the valve annulus, a scalloped ring of fibrous tissue.

## PHYSIOLOGY

The pulmonic valve opens in ventricular systole when pressure in the right ventricle exceeds that of the pulmonary artery. The valve closes at the end of systole when the pressure in the pulmonary artery is greater than in the right ventricle. Closure of the pulmonic valve produces the P2 component of the second heart sound.

## PULMONIC STENOSIS

Pulmonic stenosis involves fixed or dynamic obstruction of blood flow from the right ventricle to the pulmonary vasculature. It is mostly seen in the setting of congenital heart disease.

### ETIOLOGY

| Congenital heart disease (most common) | • Tetralogy of Fallot<br>• Transposition of great arteries<br>• Isolated valvular pulmonic stenosis<br>• Noonan syndrome (60%) with PS |
|---|---|
| Other causes (rare) | • Carcinoid syndrome<br>• Rheumatic heart disease<br>• External compression by sinus of Valsalva aneurysms, aortic graft aneurysms or large mediastinal tumors<br>• Cardiac tumors compressing RVOT |

Obstruction can arise from the subvalvular, valvular, or supravalvular regions.

• Valvular: Dysplastic, bicuspid, or unicuspid valves
• Subvalvular: Narrowing of infundibulum/RVOT, which can be seen in tetralogy of Fallot or double-chambered right ventricle, congenital VSD, severe right ventricular hypertrophy, external compression by mass or tumor
• Supravalvular: Obstruction at the level of the main pulmonary artery or its more distal branches (e.g., Noonan's syndrome and Williams syndrome) (see Fig. 11-3)

### 2D FINDINGS

• Right ventricular hypertrophy (normal thickness of the RV is <5 mm at end-diastole) (Fig. 11-1A)
• Right ventricular enlargement (Fig. 11-1B and C)
• Thickened pulmonic valve leaflets with systolic doming
• Post-stenotic dilatation of pulmonary artery

### M-MODE

• Exaggerated "a" wave of PV during diastole (due to increased force of right atrial contraction against stenotic valve)
• Right ventricular hypertrophy (best measured in subcostal view)

### PW AND CW DOPPLER

• Normally the systolic gradient across the pulmonic valve is low.

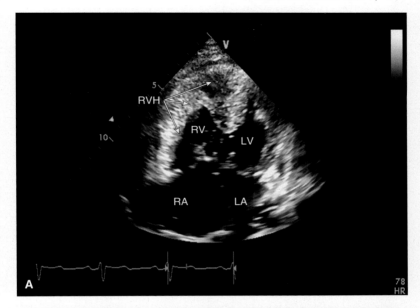

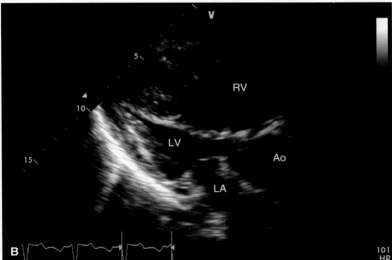

**Figure 11-1.** **(A)** A4C view from patient with AV canal defect showing massive RV hypertrophy (*arrows*). **(B)** PLAX and **(C)** PSAX views from patient with severe primary pulmonary hypertension showing marked RV dilatation and remodeling. Note in PSAX how ventricles have "swapped" shapes small crescentic, 'D-shaped' LV and thickened, spherical RV. These changes reflect marked elevation in right heart pressures. (*continued*)

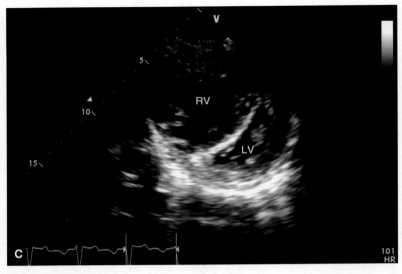

**Figure 11-1.** (*Continued*)

- Calculate peak transvalvular gradient via the modified Bernoulli equation: $\Delta P = 4v^2$ using CW Doppler. The best images are obtained in the parasternal short-axis view with the Doppler sampling parallel to flow (Fig. 11-2)
- In cases of multiple areas of stenosis, PW Doppler may be useful in determining the level of obstruction
- Pulmonary artery systolic pressure = right ventricular systolic pressure – pressure gradient across pulmonic valve
- Calculate pulmonic valve area (PVA) using continuity equation; CSA = cross sectional area. SV = stroke volume. VTI = velocity time integral (continuity equation accuracy is reduced secondary to difficulty in measuring RVOT CSA)

$$SV_{RVOT} = SV_{PA}$$
$$SV = CSA \times VTI$$
$$CSA_{RVOT} \times VTI_{RVOT} = CSA_{PA} \times VTI_{PA}$$
$$PVA = CSA_{PA} = (CSA_{RVOT} \times VTI_{RVOT})/VTI_{PA}$$

| TABLE 11-1 | Parameters for Determining Severity of Pulmonic Stenosis | |
|---|---|---|
| | **Peak gradient** | **Peak velocity** |
| **Mild PS** | <36 mmHg | <3 m/s |
| **Moderate PS** | 36–64 mmHg | 3–4 m/s |
| **Severe PS** | >64 mmHg | >4 m/s |

From Baumgartner, H, Hung J, Bermejo J, et al. Echocardiographic Assessment of Valve Stenosis: EAE/ASE Recommendations for Clinical Practice; *J Am Soc Echocardiogr.* 2009 Jan; 22(1):19–20, with permission from Elsevier.

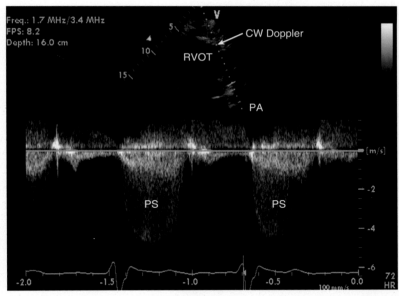

Figure 11-2. CW Doppler showing severe pulmonic stenosis with peak gradient >4 m/s.

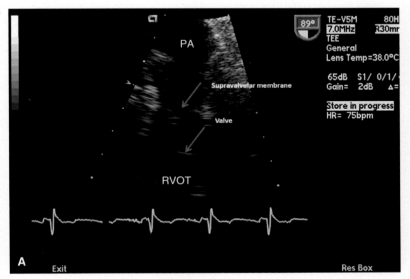

Figure 11-3. Patient with supravalvular stenosis with (A) zoomed TEE image demonstrating location of supravalvular membrane compared to the valve leaflets. (*continued*)

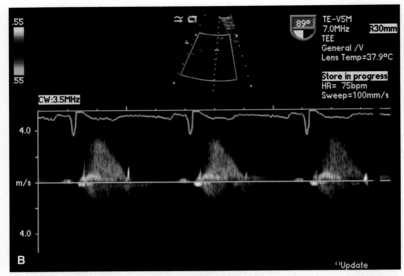

Figure 11-3. (*Continued*) (**B**) CW Doppler showing elevated gradient.

---

• **Key Point:** *Dynamic infundibular stenosis can often be distinguished from valvular stenosis as in the former scenario, the jet tends to be "dagger shaped" and late peaking in systole, indicating dynamic obstruction, whereas in valvular stenosis the jet peaks earlier in systole and does not change with hemodynamic maneuvers.*

---

## COLOR DOPPLER

- Useful in determining direction and location of stenotic jet for alignment of PW and CW Doppler
- Turbulent flow may be noted on color Doppler

## PULMONIC REGURGITATION

Pulmonic regurgitation is usually an incidental finding. Trace to mild PR is found in nearly all individuals and is usually not a pathologic finding. Pathologic PR is often found in the setting of pulmonary hypertension.

---

• **Key Point:** *Most often, significant PR is found in the setting of pulmonary hypertension.*

## ETIOLOGY

| **Pulmonary hypertension** | • Primary pulmonary hypertension<br>• Secondary pulmonary hypertension (most common cause) |
|---|---|
| **Other causes** | • Infective endocarditis (rare)<br>• Myxomatous degeneration<br>• Carcinoid heart disease (usually occurs when liver metastases present and tricuspid valve involvement)<br>• Tetralogy of Fallot (especially with a history of trans-annular patch repair)<br>• Syphilis<br>• Medications (methysergide, pergolide, fenfluramine)<br>• Marfan's syndrome<br>• Takayasu's arteritis<br>• Iatrogenic trauma from Swan–Ganz catheter or from balloon valvuloplasty or pulmonic valve surgery<br>• Congenital absence or redundancy of pulmonic valve |

## 2D FINDINGS

- RV enlargement suggestive of RV volume overload
- Enlarged RVOT, main PA
- Pulmonic valve leaflet malcopatation
- Pulmonic valve vegetations in endocarditis

## M-MODE

- Right ventricular enlargement (most often seen with chronic PR)
- Diastolic septal flattening suggests RV volume overload (not specific sign for PR).
- Premature opening of pulmonic valve (opening before QRS complex) secondary to elevated RVEDP

## CW AND PW DOPPLER

- Determine PA end-diastolic pressure using end-diastolic flow velocity of the pulmonic regurgitant jet: $\Delta P = 4v^2 + RA$ pressure
- **Dense** jet with **steep deceleration** and **early termination of diastolic flow** suggests severe PR (Fig. 11-4)
- Presystolic forward flow across the pulmonic valve suggests elevated RVEDP (Fig. 11-5)

## COLOR DOPPLER

- Should show a diastolic jet directed toward the RV beginning at the line of leaflet coaptation

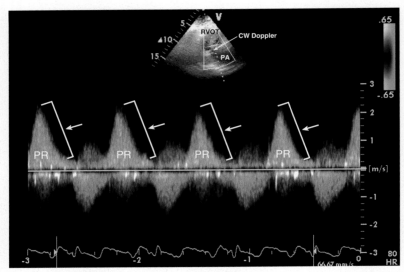

**Figure 11-4.** TTE PSAX view with CW Doppler of pulmonic valve showing dense diastolic jet with short deceleration time (*arrows*) suggestive of severe PR.

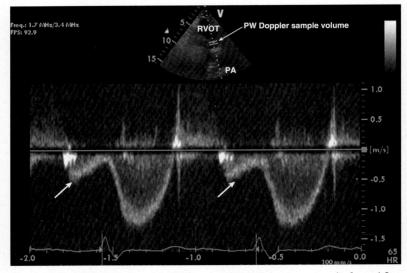

**Figure 11-5.** TTE PSAX view with PW Doppler of RVOT showing presystolic forward flow (*arrows*) due to premature equalization of RV and PA pressures in diastole. This can be seen in severe PR with premature opening of the pulmonic valve.

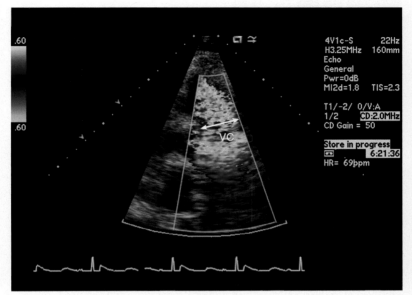

**Figure 11-6.** Color Doppler of RVOT showing a wide vena contracta associated with severe PR.

- The width of the jet is narrow in mild pulmonic regurgitation and arises at the valve commissure with a narrow vena contracta
- As the PR gets worse, the **width of the jet increases** and can fill the RVOT (Fig. 11-6)

---

- **Key Point:** *Color Doppler jet of severe PR may be brief secondary to rapid equilibration of RV and pulmonary pressures. Therefore always review spectral Doppler as severe PR can be missed when looking at color Doppler alone!*

---

# 12

# Tricuspid Valve Disorders

Daniel H. Cooper and Thomas K. Kurian

## HIGH-YIELD FINDINGS

### Severe tricuspid regurgitation
- Vena contracta width >0.7 cm
- RA area occupied by tricuspid regurgitation (TR) jet ≥40%
- Gross leaflet malcoaptation
- TV annulus dilatation >4 cm
- Dense, early peaking TR CW Doppler envelope
- Hepatic vein systolic flow reversal
- RA/RV enlargement
- Evidence of RV volume overload

### Severe tricuspid stenosis
- Leaflets thickened, calcified, fused, immobile
- Diastolic leaflet doming
- RA enlargement
- Elevated TV peak inflow velocity >1 m/s
- Mean TV gradient >7 mmHg
- Pressure half time >190 ms

## KEY VIEWS
- Parasternal RV inflow tract (RVIT)
- Parasternal short-axis RV inflow/outflow
- Apical four chamber
- Subcostal four chamber

## TRICUSPID REGURGITATION

### General Principles
- TR is common. Some degree of TR is found in nearly 80% to 90% of the population.
- **Primary valvular causes** of TR include Ebstein's anomaly (see Chapter 17), carcinoid (see Chapter 19), endocarditis (see Chapter 14), myxomatous degeneration, and rheumatic disease. **Secondary causes** include any process that leads to tricuspid annulus dilatation due to right ventricular and/or right atrial enlargement (e.g.,

**Pulmonary hypertension,** left ventricular dysfunction, left-to-right shunts, right ventricular infarction).
- Mild TR in general is benign. Moderate to severe TR is associated with reduced long-term survival, even in the absence of comorbid pulmonary hypertension or ventricular dysfunction.

## Assessment of TR by Transthoracic Echocardiography (TTE)

*General Principles*
- The tricuspid valve (TV) consists of three, anatomically distinct leaflets (anterior, posterior, septal).
- These leaflets are thinner and have an annulus that is larger than the mitral valve. **The valve is more apically displaced in location compared to the mitral valve and is not in direct continuity with the pulmonic valve.**

---

- **Key Point:** *The atrio-ventricular (AV) valves are always associated with their respective ventricle. The relative position of the AV valves has important ramifications. In patients with congenital heart disease where the ventricular position may be altered the RV may be recognized by the more apically displaced TV. An AV canal defect is recognized by the AV valves being on the **same** plane. Ebstein's anomaly is recognized by the septal tricuspid leaflet being markedly apically displaced.*

---

- The TV sits anterior and rightward of the mitral valve. It is separated from the pulmonic valve by the infundibulum.

---

- **Key Point:** *This is in contrast to the left heart where there is no infundibulum and the mitral and aortic valves are separated only by a fibrous continuum. This has ramifications for the effects of mitral and aortic valvular pathology such as endocarditis, which can spread to either valve causing annular or aortic root abscess.*

---

## 2D ECHOCARDIOGRAM

- In general, tricuspid leaflet **location, thickness, mobility, and coaptation** should be assessed in all available views.
  - The **RVIT** is the one view where the **posterior leaflet** is seen along with the anterior leaflet, otherwise in the parasternal short-axis and apical four-chamber view the anterior and septal leaflets are seen (see Fig. 12-1A).
  - With Ebstein's anomaly there is (a) apical displacement ($>0.8$ cm/m$^2$) of the septal leaflet, (b) a large, "sail-like" anterior leaflet with a variable number of tethering attachments to the anterior RV free wall, and (c) atrialization of the RV secondary to apically displaced TV coaptation (see Fig. 12-1B). The size of the RV that remains unaffected is a major determinant of prognosis.
  - Rheumatic disease of the TV produces thickened chordae progressing to leaflet tip thickening/fusion and restricted movement. **It is rarely seen in the absence of mitral valve involvement.**
  - Carcinoid tumors cause a serotonin-induced fibrosis that results in short, thickened, and restricted tricuspid leaflets that are **"club"**-like in appearance and fixed in an open position (see Fig. 12-4).

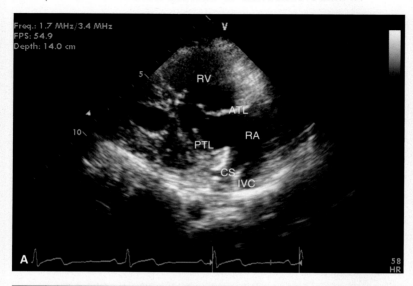

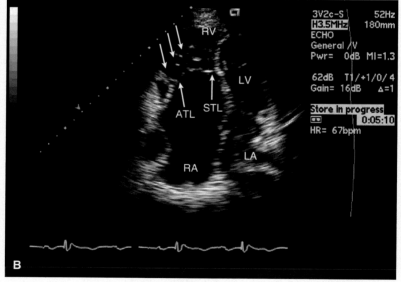

**Figure 12-1. A:** RVIT view showing posterior and anterior TV leaflets in patient without TV disease. **B:** A4C showing apically displaced septal leaflet and long, "sail"-like anterior leaflet tethered to the RV free wall (*arrows*), in patient with Ebstein's anomaly.

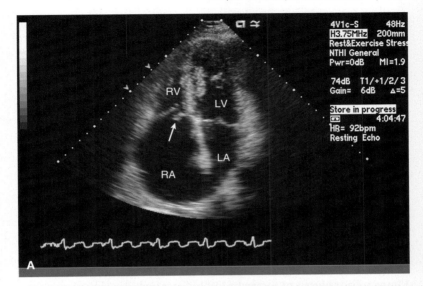

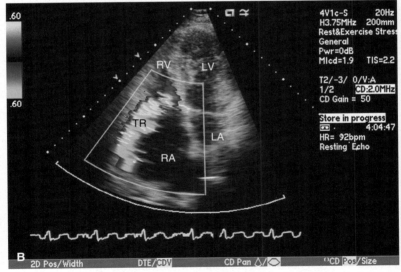

Figure 12-2. (A) A4C chamber view both with and without color Doppler acquired from cardiac transplant patient (bi-atrial elongation because of atrial anastomoses). A flail septal leaflet of the tricuspid valve (*arrow*) is seen with (B) consequent severe eccentric TR as a complication of cardiac biopsy. Typical of a flail leaflet the jet is directed to the opposite side from the affected leaflet.

> • **Key Point:** *The serotonin-like substance is deactivated in the pulmonary circulation therefore right-sided valves are only typically affected. However left sided valves may also be involved in the presence of an interatrial shunt with right to left flow. Carcinoid TV disease is a **primary** valve problem and is differentiated from TV tethering, from general RV dilatation, where the valve leaflets are normal.*

- Flail leaflets can be seen in the setting of endocarditis, repeated endomyocardial biopsies (e.g., heart transplant patients), myxomatous degeneration, and blunt chest trauma (Fig. 12-2).
- **Chamber dimensions and biventricular function**
  - RA and RV enlargement are common in severe TR.
  - TV annulus dilatation >4 cm is often seen in severe TR unless it is acute.
  - RV systolic function can be compromised in the setting of pulmonary hypertension, left ventricular failure, and RV infarction.
- **Interventricular septum**
  - Paradoxical septal motion with **diastolic flattening** is seen in RV *volume* overload
  - RV *pressure* overload may eventually develop causing a "D-shaped" LV due to flattening of the septum in both systole and diastole
- **Inferior vena cava (IVC) dilatation (>2.1 cm)** may be seen in severe TR.
- **Intracardiac catheters or pacemaker/defibrillator leads** should be noted for vegetations (endocarditis) or promoting leaflet malcopatation.

## COLOR DOPPLER

- The **RA area occupied by the TR regurgitant jet** and **vena contracta width** are the most commonly utilized methods to estimate TR severity.
  - Severe TR: Regurgitant jet area **≥40%** of RA area and vena contracta width **≥0.7 mm** (Fig. 12-3)
- **PISA method** (not commonly used)
  - Severe TR: PISA radius >10 mm for a Nyquist limit of 30 cm/s (or >7 mm for 40 cm/s).
  - Severe TR: EROA ≥0.4 cm$^2$ and regurgitant volume ≥45 mL/beat.

## PULSED- AND CONTINUOUS-WAVE DOPPLER

- **Density** of the continuous-wave (CW) TR envelope correlates with TR severity.
  - Severe TR: TR envelope as **dense** as TV inflow and is **early peaking** because of rapid equilibration of pressures between RA and RV (Fig. 12-3).
- **Elevated TV inflow velocity (>1.0 m/s)** is seen in severe TR.
- **Pulsed wave (PW) of the hepatic vein flow (subcostal view):**
  - Normal or mild TR: Systolic predominance
  - Moderate TR: Systolic blunting
  - Severe TR: **Systolic flow reversal**
- **Estimated pulmonary artery systolic pressure (PASP)**
  - CW Doppler of TR: (modified Bernoulli equation) $4v^2$ + mean RAP

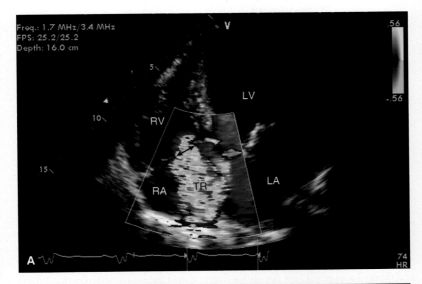

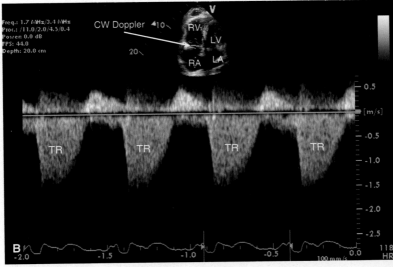

**Figure 12-3. A:** A4C view with severe TR, seen on color Doppler with wide vena contracta (*arrow*) and jet filling a large portion of the RA. **B:** Spectral Doppler of TR showing early peaking, low velocity, dense Doppler envelope.

- **Key Point:** *When TR is severe it is difficult to accurately estimate mean RAP and therefore PASP.*

## Other Considerations

- If RV pressure is elevated, the TR jet will be more impressive on color Doppler than a similar regurgitant volume in patients without pressure overload.
- Chamber sizes, biventricular function, interventricular septal motion, estimated PASP, and leaflet morphology will aid in differentiating between the etiologies listed above.
- Detailed TV assessment is particularly important in patients with comorbid MV disease.
  - To optimize outcomes, MV intervention for severe MS or MR should take place before severe TR, RV dysfunction, or congestive heart failure develops.
  - TV annuloplasty should be considered at the time of MV surgery for patients with a dilated RV annulus and severe TR.

## TRICUSPID STENOSIS

### General Principles

- Tricuspid stenosis (TS) is rare and is almost always associated with rheumatic heart disease. It is extremely rare to find in isolation (i.e., in the absence of mitral or aortic valve disease).
  - Less common causes: Congenital abnormalities, endocarditis, carcinoid and large RA masses that may mimic TS (Fig. 12-4).

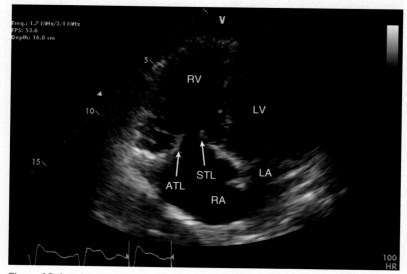

**Figure 12-4.** A4C, "RV-focused" view showing thickened, "club-like" septal and anterior tricuspid valve leaflets fixed in an open position. This appearance is suggestive of Carcinoid disease.

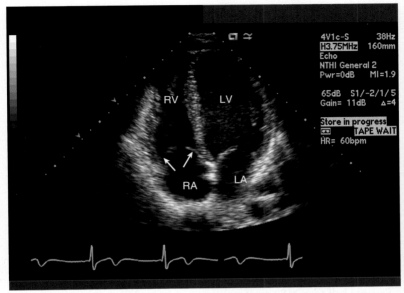

**Figure 12-5.** Doming of the tricuspid valve (*arrows*) suggestive of rheumatic tricuspid stenosis.

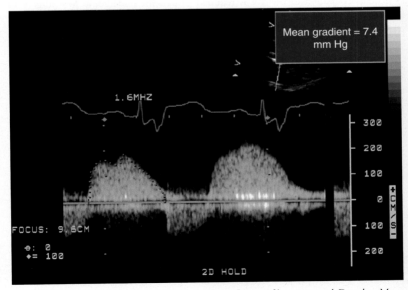

**Figure 12-6.** Tricuspid stenosis with dense, flat inflow profile on spectral Doppler. Mean gradient is markedly elevated (~7.4 mmHg).

## Assessment of TS by TTE

### 2D ECHOCARDIOGRAPHY

- **Leaflet/chordae morphology and mobility**
  - Leaflet thickening, fusion of the commissures, and retraction and thickening of the subvalvular apparatus are features of rheumatic heart disease.
  - Diastolic "doming" of the leaflets is characteristic of rheumatic TS (Fig. 12-5).
- **Chamber dimensions**
  - RA enlargement is common in severe TS
- **IVC dilatation** may also be seen in severe TS

### M-MODE

- **Reduced E-F slope** reflects the restricted leaflet motion in TS

### DOPPLER

- **Elevated TV inflow velocity >1 m/s** (Fig. 12-6)
- **Mean TV gradient:**
  - Normal: 2 mmHg; Moderate 2 to 5 mmHg; Severe ≥5 mmHg
- **Pressure half time ≥190 ms** is consistent with severe TR

### Other Considerations

- Careful evaluation of the TV is required in patients undergoing MV surgery to exclude the need for TV repair as it may be subtle and overlooked, especially if adequate images are not obtained for interpretation.

# 13 Evaluation of Prosthetic Valves

Jose A. Madrazo

## HIGH-YIELD CONCEPTS

- Whenever possible, know the type, size, and age of the prosthesis being evaluated.
- Serial echocardiographic evaluation of prosthetic valves should be referenced to a **baseline study** performed early after implantation.
- High gradients across a valve may be due to:
  - Valve dysfunction/obstruction
  - Increased flow:
    - Regurgitation
    - High output states
  - Patient-prosthesis mismatch
- The ultrasound beam cannot penetrate the dense material of prosthetic valves. **Multiple views** are required to allow the beam to interrogate chambers without interference from prosthesis-related artifact. **In patients with multiple prosthetic valves, TEE is often necessary** if clinical suspicion of prosthetic valve dysfunction is high.

## KEY POINTS

- The following should raise concern for **severe** prosthesis malfunction:
  - **Aortic** valves:
    - Stenosis
      - Peak velocity >4 m/s
      - Mean gradient >35 mmHg
      - LVOT/AoV velocity or VTI ratio <0.25
      - Aortic acceleration time >100 ms (rounded velocity contour)
    - Regurgitation
      - Regurgitant jet width ≥65% of LVOT (at Nyquist limit = 50 to 60 cm/s)
      - Dense regurgitant jet with PHT <200 ms
      - Regurgitant volume >60 mL/beat; regurgitant fraction >50%
      - LVOT TVI >> RVOT TVI
      - Prominent holodiastolic flow reversal in the descending aorta
  - **Mitral** valves:
    - Stenosis
      - Peak velocity ≥2.5 m/s
      - Mean gradient >10 mmHg
      - MV inflow PHT >200 ms

- ○ Regurgitation
  - Dense early, peaking jet (triangular)
  - EROA ≥0.5 cm$^2$
  - Regurgitant jet of ≥8 cm$^2$ area
  - Vena contracta ≥0.6 cm
  - Regurgitant volume ≥60 mL/beat; regurgitant fraction >50%
  - Pulmonary vein systolic flow reversal in one or more veins
  - MV/LVOT TVI ratio >2.5

- The echocardiographic evaluation of prosthetic valves is a challenging task as there are many different types of prostheses and they frequently impart imaging artifacts and shadowing (Fig. 13-1).
- Understanding the types of valves available helps determine the expected appearance, gradients, and physiologic regurgitation.
- Valves are generally divided into bioprosthetic or mechanical.
  - Bioprosthetic valves may be stented (higher profile), stentless, homografts, or heterografts.
  - Mechanical valves may be ball-cage or tilting disk (single or double).

## REGURGITATION

- Most mechanical valves will have some built in **"physiologic" regurgitation** (Fig. 13-2). Knowing the type of valve will help determine the expected pattern of regurgitation. Some common examples:
  - Bileaflet tilting disk valves will have two small lateral (and one small central for St. Jude's) jets of regurgitation that are angled inward.
  - Single tilting disk valves will have a central area of regurgitation around the hinge-point (that is larger than what is seen in bileaflet valves).
- Perivalvular leak (typically unilateral, eccentric, turbulent jet) is in contrast **pathologic** (Fig. 13-3) and occurs most often in redo valve replacement surgery or when extensive calcium debridement is required prior to valve implantation (newer percutaneously inserted valves will not uncommonly have a small perivalvular regurgitant jet).

---

- **Key Point:** *In general "physiologic" regurgitation* **extends <1 to 2 cm from the valve, is symmetrical and low velocity (i.e., not turbulent).**

---

- Start your evaluation by identifying the valve and confirming the expected appearance. Look for **stability** of the valve and ring. Excessive movement of the entire prosthesis ("**rocking**") suggests dehiscence. Evaluate leaflet/disk motion when they are visible. Pay attention to the presence of calcifications, thrombi, or vegetations.

---

- **Key Point:** *Unlike native valve endocarditis, prosthetic valve infection usually begins where the sewing ring meets the annulus and then spreads to the valve leaflets.*

---

- Prosthetic valves will cause shadowing distal to the ultrasound beam and make those areas difficult to inspect visually. Standard and off-axis views should be selected to **interrogate areas of interest first and then the prosthesis to minimize shadowing** (e.g., for evaluating MR for a mitral prosthesis the PLAX and subcostal images can visualize the LA without significant artifact compared to the apical four-chamber view). TEE is often necessary when clinical suspicion of prosthetic valve dysfunction is high especially when multiple prostheses are present (Fig. 13-4).

Diastole                    Systole

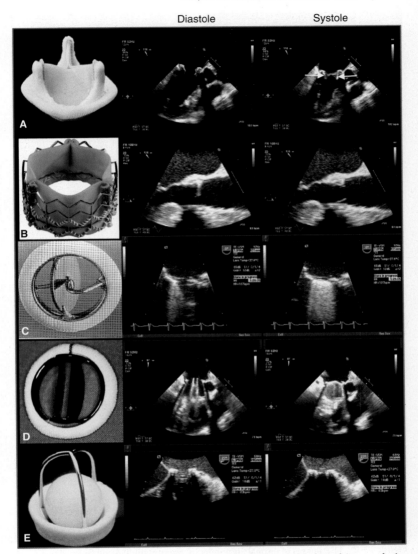

Figure 13-1. **TEE images of prosthetic valve types and transesophageal images during diastole and systole. A:** Bioprosthesis in the mitral position. Note the prominent struts (*arrows*). **B:** Edwards SAPIEN transcathether aortic valve. (From Baim DS, *Grossman's Cardiac Catheterization, Angiography, and Intervention, Seventh Edition.* Philadelphia: Lippincott Williams & Wilkins, 2006.) **C:** Single tilting disk valve. (From Weyman AE. *Principles and Practice of Echocardiography. 2nd ed.* Philadelphia: Lea & Febiger; 1994.) **D:** Bileaflet tilting disk valve. **E:** Ball and cage valve.

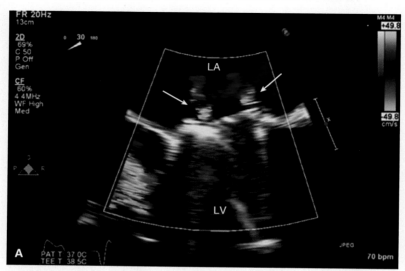

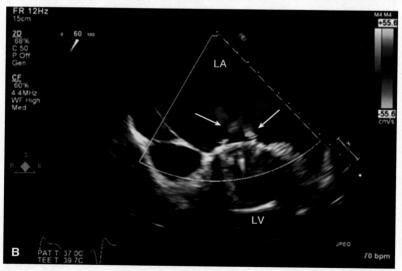

**Figure 13-2. TEE images of normal "physiologic" regurgitation. A** and **B:** Small peripheral regurgitant jets in bileaflet tilting disk valve (*arrows*).

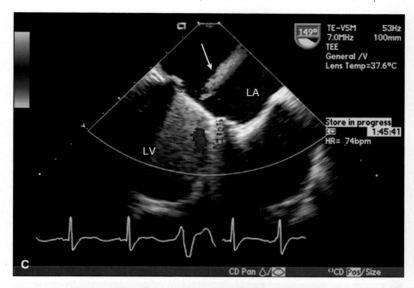

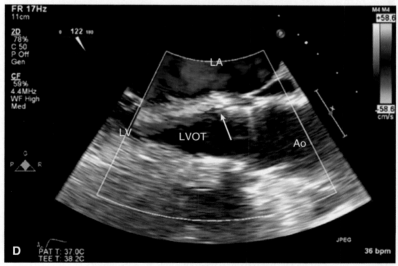

**Figure 13-2.** (*Continued*) **C:** Larger central jet in single tilting disk valve (*arrow*). **D:** Mild paravalvular regurgitation in Edwards SAPIEN percutaneously implanted valve (*arrow*).

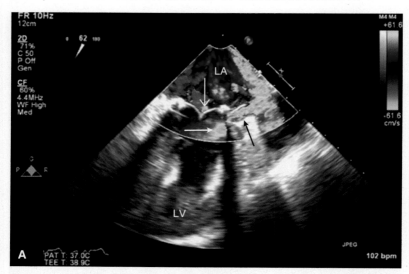

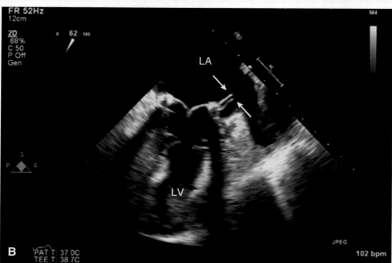

**Figure 13-3. Pathologic paravalvular regurgitation. A:** TEE images at 60 degrees of a bioprosthetic valve in the mitral position demonstrating severe perialvular regurgitation (*black arrow*) and mild "physiologic" central regurgitation (*open white arrow*). Note the area of flow convergence (PISA) on the ventricular side (*solid white arrow*). **B:** Suture dehiscence clearly seen (*white arrows*).

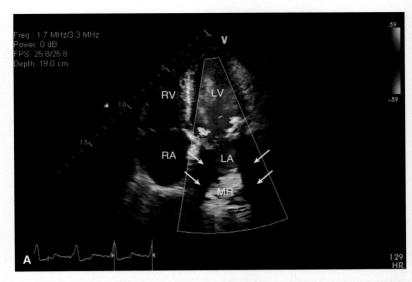

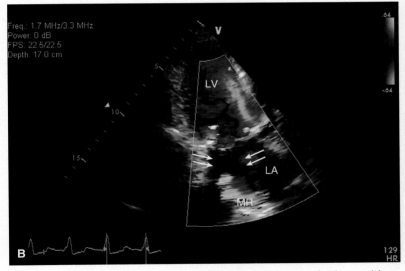

**Figure 13-4. Severe perivalvular mitral regurgitation can be missed.** Ultrasound beam attenuation artifact (*arrows*) allows only distal segments of the MR jet to be visualized in these **(A)** AP4 and **(B)** APLAX images. (*continued*)

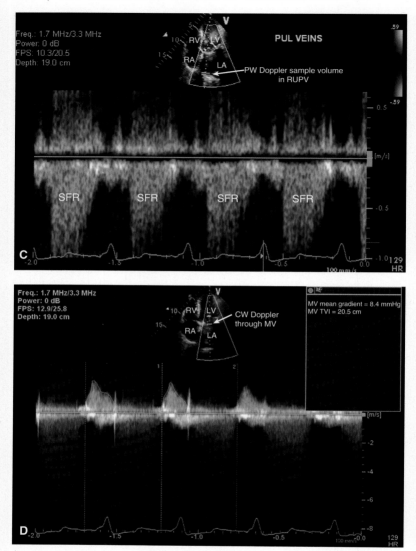

**Figure 13-4.** (*Continued*) The MR jet reaches to the back of the LA with (**C**) pulmonary vein systolic flow reversal, elevated mean mitral gradient (**D**)

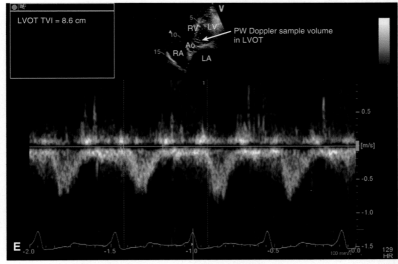

**Figure 13-4.** (*Continued*) and an MV TVI that is close to 2.5 times the measured LVOT TVI (**E**) which is consistent with severe MR.

- In addition to TEE traditional fluoroscopy or gated CT scanning can be used to assess leaflet opening and closure angles with mechanical disk valves. Pannus (exuberant scar formation) or thrombus may impair valve disk motion and lead to pathologic obstruction and regurgitation.
- On color Doppler:
  - Look for flow pattern and velocity during the open phase of the valve. Flow convergence with aliasing may be the first clue that the valve is stenosed or there is increased flow through it.
  - Assess for regurgitation during the closed phase of the valve. Pay attention to the origin and direction of regurgitant leaks if present. An area of flow convergence on the opposite surface of the valve (e.g., LV surface of MV prosthesis) is always abnormal and may be the only clear sign of perivalvular leak (Fig. 13-5).

## HIGH GRADIENTS

- It is important to know the type of valve a patient has as well as its size. This will dictate the expected effective orifice area (EOA) and gradients for that valve. There are tables that can be referenced in order to know these expected values. The EOA should preferably be indexed to body surface area (EOAi). The age of the valve since implantation can help predict clinical complications (bioprosthetic valves tend to degenerate earlier than mechanical valves and pannus formation can occur in older valves of either type, especially in the aortic position). A general guide for expected gradients for prosthetic valves in the aortic and mitral positions are given with more detailed tables available in the literature. It is however a better strategy, to compare findings to the baseline Doppler derived gradients and valve area performed soon after valve implantation (Table 13-1).

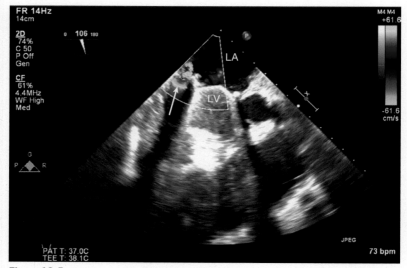

**Figure 13-5. Severe perivalvular mitral regurgitation can be missed.** TEE view showing an area of flow convergence with aliasing on the ventricular surface (*arrow*) of a bileaflet tilting disk valve in the mitral position in a patient with severe regurgitation.

---

- **Key Point:** *If prior echocardiograms are available be sure to know what the gradients were in the past and always compare the current measurements to these when possible. An increase in gradient over time should raise suspicion for prosthesis malfunction.*

---

- An increased gradient across a valve may be the only clue that a problem exists. A high gradient may be observed as a result of stenosis (valvular or subvalvular), increased flow across the valve (such as in significant regurgitation or a hyperdynamic state), or technical aspects (such as incorrect PW Doppler location and measurement).

- All valves are **inherently stenotic** compared to native valves. At its extreme, a valve may be too small compared to the patient's body surface area and hemodynamic requirements, known as *patient prosthesis mismatch* (PPM). **PPM is severe when EOAi <0.65 cm²/m² for the aortic valve or <1.2 cm²/m² for the mitral valve.** As a result, there may be an increased gradient across the valve due to an increased stroke volume across a fixed orifice even when the prosthesis is normally functioning. This has ramifications for resolution of left ventricular hypertrophy (aortic valve PPM) and pulmonary hypertension (mitral valve PPM) and the associated morbidity and mortality of these conditions.

- Another important concept that may be clinically important in patients with prosthetic valves is that of pressure recovery. According to Bernoulli's principle, as the flow of a fluid accelerates toward a narrowing, there is a loss of pressure (the fluid gains kinetic energy but loses pressure energy). As the fluid moves distal to the narrowing it slows down and regains some of that lost pressure energy and this is called *pressure recovery phenomenon.* Thus, the Doppler measured peak instantaneous gradient may be significantly higher than one measured by cardiac catheterization (where the sampling is performed in the aorta after pressure has recovered). Pressure

| TABLE 13-1 | Expected Values for Normally Functioning Aortic and Mitral Prosthetic Valves | | |
|---|---|---|---|
| Valve type | Peak velocity (m/sec) | Peak gradient (mmHg) | Mean gradient (mmHg) |
| Aortic position | | | |
| St. Jude | $2.3 \pm 0.6$ | $22 \pm 12$ | $12 \pm 7$ |
| Bjork–Shiley | $2.6 \pm 0.5$ | $27 \pm 9$ | $14 \pm 6$ |
| Starr–Edwards | $3.2 \pm 0.2$ | $40 \pm 3$ | $24 \pm 4$ |
| Tissue | $2.1 \pm 0.5$ | $19 \pm 9$ | $11 \pm 5$ |
| Mitral position | | | |
| St. Jude | $1.6 \pm 0.3$ | $11 \pm 4.0$ | $5 \pm 2.0$ |
| Bjork–Shiley | $1.6 \pm 0.3$ | $10 \pm 3$ | $5 \pm 2$ |
| Starr–Edwards | $1.8 \pm 0.4$ | $13 \pm 5$ | $5 \pm 2$ |
| Beall | $1.8 \pm 0.2$ | $13 \pm 4$ | $6 \pm 2$ |
| Tissue | $1.5 \pm 0.3$ | $9.9 \pm 3.4$ | $4.8 \pm 1.7$ |

Adapted from Nanda NC, Cooper JW, Mahan EF, et al. Echo-cardiographic assessment of prosthetic valves. *Circulation*. 1991;84(Suppl 1):228–239, with permission.

recovery is most pronounced with higher velocities through small bi-leaflet mechanical valves (such as 19 mm valves) in patients with small aortas (diameter ≤3 cm) where laminar flow is preserved. This discrepancy is exacerbated as CW Doppler may measure **localized high velocities** within the mechanical bi-leaflet valve (side orifices are smaller than the central orifice) with the resultant instantaneous gradient not being a true reflection of the overall gradient between the aorta and LV.

- **Key Point:** *When comparing gradients obtained by cardiac catheterization versus echocardiography it is best to use **mean gradients**. Peak pressure gradients most commonly reported after cardiac catheterization use the "peak-to-peak" pressure difference between the LV and aorta which is different and always lower than the **instantaneous** pressure difference between the LV and aorta measured by Doppler echocardiography (Fig. 13-6).*

- **Key Point:** *Both valvular stenosis and regurgitation will result in increased gradients across a valve. However, stenosis will generally result in maintenance of a transvalvular gradient for a longer period of time. Thus, stenosed mitral valves have an increased pressure half-time (PHT); similarly, stenosed aortic valves have an increased time to peak acceleration (acceleration time, AT) (Fig. 13-7). **Elevated gradients with normal AT or PHT are suggestive of regurgitation, high flow states, PPM, or technical aspects like pressure recovery rather than valvular obstruction.***

- Using the principles discussed, a systematic approach for assessing high gradients for prosthetic valves in the aortic (Fig 13-8) as well mitral (Table 13-2) position has been provided by the American Society of Echocardiography guidelines.

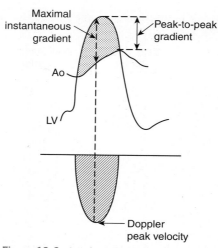

**Figure 13-6.** Simultaneous pressure tracings from the LV and aorta invasively measured compared to Doppler derived pressure gradients.

| Increased gradient due to: | High flow/normal valve | Valve stenosis |
|---|---|---|
| Mitral Doppler | 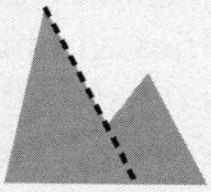 | 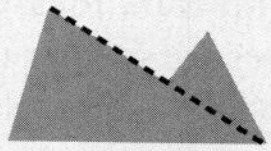 |
| Pressure half-time (PHT) | Normal (<130 ms) | Increased (>than 200 ms) |
| Aortic Doppler | 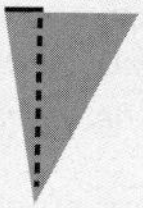 | 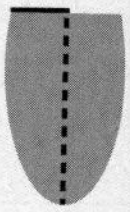 |
| Acceleration time (AT): | Normal (<100 ms) Triangular | Increased (>100 ms) Rounded contour |

**Figure 13-7. Doppler profiles of prosthetic valves with elevated gradients due to high flow versus stenosis.**

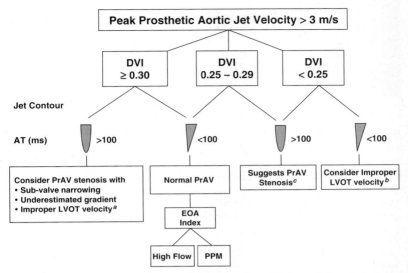

Figure 13-8. **Algorithm for evaluation of elevated peak prosthetic aortic jet velocity** incorporating DVI, jet contour, and AT.
[a]PW Doppler sample too close to the valve (particularly when jet velocity by CW Doppler is ≥4 m/s).
[b]PW Doppler sample too far (apical) from the valve (particularly when jet velocity is 3–3.9 m/s).
[c]Stenosis further substantiated by EOA derivation compared with reference values if valve type and size are known. Fluoroscopy and TEE are helpful for further assessment, particularly in bileaflet valves. AVR, aortic valve replacement. (Adapted from Zoghbi, Chambers JB, Dumesnil JG, et al. Recommendations for evaluation of prosthetic valves with echocardiography and Doppler ultrasound. *J Am Soc Echocardiogr.* 2009; (9): 975–1014).

| TABLE 13-2 | Expected Parameters for a Normal Mitral Valve Prosthesis and Parameters Suggesting Possible or Significant Stenosis | | |
|---|---|---|---|
| | Normal[a] | Possible stenosis[c] | Suggests significant stenosis[a,c] |
| Peak velocity (m/s)[b,d] | <1.9 | 1.9–2.5 | ≥2.5 |
| Mean gradient (mmHg)[b,d] | ≤5 | 6–10 | >10 |
| $VTI_{prMV}/VTI_{Lvo}$[b,d] | <2.2 | 2.2–2.5 | >2.5 |
| EOA (cm²) | ≥2.0 | 1–2 | <1 |
| PHT (ms) | <130 | 130–200 | >200 |

[a]Best specificity for normality or abnormality is seen if the majority of the parameters listed are normal or abnormal, respectively.
[b]Slightly higher cutoff values than shown may be seen in some bioprosthetic valves.
[c]Values of the parameters should prompt a closer evaluation of valve function and/or other considerations such as increased flow, increased heart rate, or PPM.
[d]These parameters are also abnormal in the presence of significant prosthetic MR.
*PHT,* pressure half-time; *PrMV,* prosthetic mitral valve.
(From Zoghbi WA, Chambers JB, Dumesnil JG, et al. Recommendations for evaluation of prosthetic valves with echocardiography and Doppler ultrasound. *J Am Soc Echocardiogr.* 2009;22(9): 975–1014, with permission from Elsevier.)

# 14

# Infective Endocarditis

Mohammed K. Saghir, Sudeshna Banerjee,
and Daniel H. Cooper

## HIGH-YIELD FINDINGS

- The clinical presentation should always be considered when interpreting the description of valvular and annular masses on echocardiography.
- When the clinical suspicion for endocarditis is high, a TEE is the test of choice.
- Concurrent mitral and aortic valve infection is common as they are in direct continuity separated only by a fibrous band of tissue. Therefore examine the aortic root carefully for abscess.
- Vegetations often have an echodensity similar to tissue, demonstrate independent movement, and have a predilection for the leading edge and lower pressure side of native valve leaflets.
- It is uncommon not to have associated valvular regurgitation in the presence of "vegetations." Consider other possible causes of valvular masses in this situation.
- Endocarditis involving native valves often arises from the leaflets whereas endocarditis of prosthetic valves often arises where the sewing ring and annulus meets.

Infective endocarditis (IE) describes a microbial infection of the endothelial surface of the heart. Valvular involvement is common and characterized by the presence of **vegetations**. Complications include, but are not limited to, valvular insufficiency, myocardial abscess formation, pericardial effusion, arrhythmia, embolic phenomenon, and congestive heart failure. Factors that predispose a patient to IE include structural abnormality of a heart valve (e.g., bicuspid aortic valve), ventricular septal defect, prosthetic cardiac valve, age, IV drug use, hemodialysis, diabetes, and poor dental hygiene.

IE remains a clinical diagnosis and therefore persistently positive blood cultures, presence of intravascular catheters, pacemakers, physical examination, and history must be taken into account. The DUKE criteria for endocarditis seek to address this point with echocardiography providing evidence of endocardial involvement (a major criterion) if any of the following exist:

1. Presence of vegetation (tissue-like echodensity with independent motion implanted on the valve, prosthetic material, or endocardium in the trajectory of a regurgitant jet in the absence of alternative anatomic explanation)
2. Presence of abscesses
3. New dehiscence of a valve prosthesis
4. New valvular regurgitation

## TRANSTHORACIC VERSUS TRANSESOPHAGEAL ECHOCARDIOGRAPHY

- TTE remains an excellent initial diagnostic test for evaluation of intermediate risk patients for IE (Fig. 14-1). However:
  - TTE has lower resolution than TEE and can miss vegetations <0.5 cm in size.
  - Sensitivity of TTE for IE ranges from 40% to 63% with a specificity of 90% to 98%.
  - If IE is diagnosed with TTE, it should be followed by TEE to evaluate other valves and complications of IE such as abscess, fistula formation, mycotic aneurysm, pseudoaneursym, and leaflet perforations.
- TEE is the preferred initial study in high-risk patients by Duke criteria, or in patients who are poor candidates for TTE.
  - High-risk patients are defined as those with prosthetic heart valves, congenital heart disease, previous endocarditis, new murmur, heart failure, or stigmata of IE.
  - Proximity of a high frequency TEE probe to the heart allows excellent visualization of the base of the heart and aorta. The aortic and mitral valves are especially well seen.
  - Sensitivity of TEE for IE is 90% to 99% with a specificity of 91% to 99%.
  - In patients with a strong suspicion of IE and negative TEE, a repeat TEE 7 to 10 days may be considered to reassess for vegetations.

## VEGETATION

- Vegetations from IE are often a mixture of microorganisms, inflammatory cells, platelets, and fibrin.
- They are often found on the leading edge of the affected native valve on the lower pressure side or grow from the annulus if a prosthetic valve is present.
- **Because of leaflet malcoaptation or destruction, valvular regurgitation is almost always an accompanying feature** (Fig. 14-2).

> - **Key Point:** *Consider alternative diagnoses for masses that appear close to a heart valve but are not associated with valvular regurgitation; for example, a partially visualized myxoma growing from the interatrial septum to the valve (Fig. 14-3).*

- Vegetations may also be seen where regurgitant or fistula flow strikes the endocardial wall, so called "jet vegetations."
- Occasionally, vegetations can cause obstruction and mimic valvular stenosis.
- Echocardiographic images should be captured with attention to the following:
  - Presence, size, shape, and location of vegetations
  - Valvular hemodynamics
    - Carefully assess the entire valve to find regurgitant jets
    - Maximize color Doppler frame rate by reducing the Doppler window
    - Assess for evidence of volume overload or associated signs of regurgitation severity (e.g., holodiastolic flow reversal in descending aorta in patients with severe AR)
  - Examine the valvular integrity. Perforation may manifest as multiple jets with turbulence seen on the high-pressure surface of the valve leaflet (Fig. 14-4)
- Pacing wires and catheters should also be carefully inspected for vegetations (Fig. 14-5). TEE is preferred to visualize lead infections and also to determine whether the tricuspid valve is affected because of lead artifact.

> - **Key Point:** *If the regurgitant jet of an infected valve strikes the endocardial wall, that area should be closely inspected for further vegetations.*

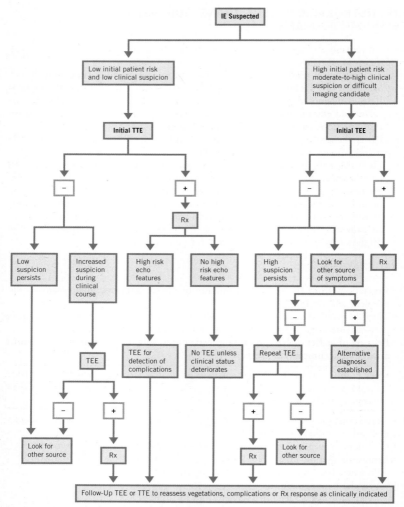

**Figure 14-1.** Algorithm for use of TTE in evaluation of patient suspected of infective endocarditis (IE). (From AHA Scientific Statement: Infective Endocarditis: Diagnosis, antimicrobial therapy, and management of complications: A statement for healthcare professionals from the Committee on Rheumatic Fever, Endocarditis, and Kawasaki Disease, Council on Cardiovascular Disease in the Young, and the Councils on Clinical Cardiology, Stroke, and Cardiovascular Surgery and Anesthesia, American Heart Association: Endorsed by the Infectious Diseases Society of America. *Circulation.* 2005;111:e394–e434.)

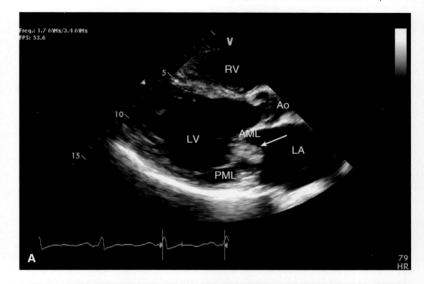

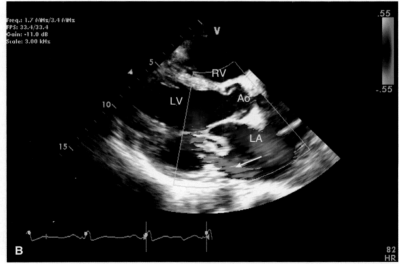

Figure 14-2. **A:** PLAX with mass seen on atrial surface of the anterior mitral leaflet consistent with vegetation (*arrow*). **B:** This causes MV malcoaptation and moderate-severe posteriorly directed MR (*arrow*).

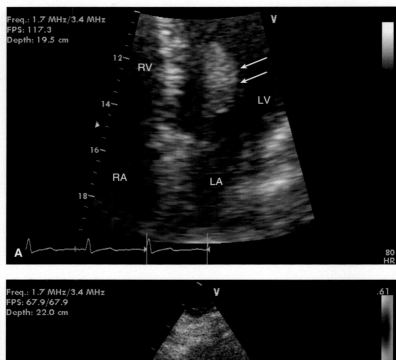

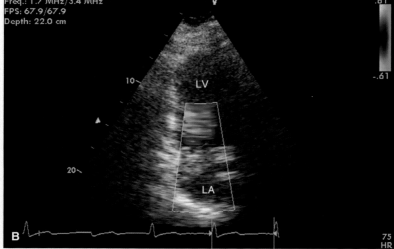

**Figure 14-3. A:** AP4 with zoomed view of MV shows mass (*arrows*) that appears to be attached to the anterior mitral leaflet (AML) suggestive of vegetation. **B:** However AP2 color Doppler shows no associated MR.

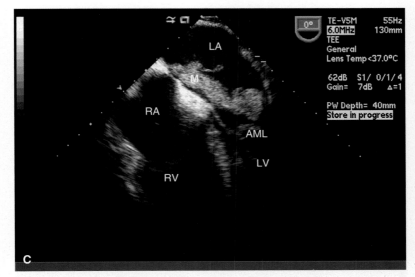

**Figure 14-3.** (*Continued*) **C:** TEE performed in same patient shows that the mass is in fact larger than appreciated on TTE and is attached to the inter-atrial septum projecting into the mitral orifice. The diagnosis of LA myxoma (M) was confirmed on pathology.

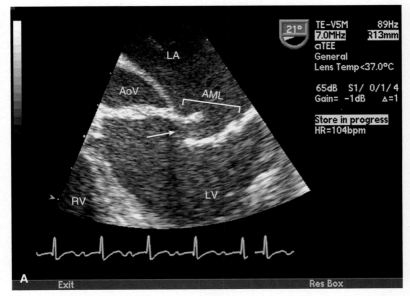

**Figure 14-4.** **A:** TEE "superior" home view zoomed on anterior mitral leaflet. There is an area of discontinuity suggestive of perforation (*arrow*). (*continued*)

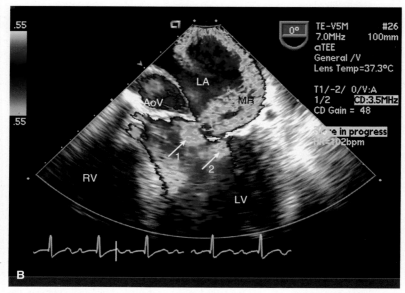

**Figure 14-4.** (*Continued*) **B:** This is confirmed on color Doppler where a separate flow acceleration and MR jet is seen (*arrow-1*) in addition to the jet that occurs at leaflet coaptation (*arrow-2*).

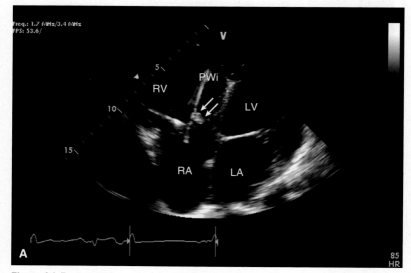

**Figure 14-5. A:** A4C focused on the RV shows pacing wire (PWi) with small vegetation near the TV (*arrows*).

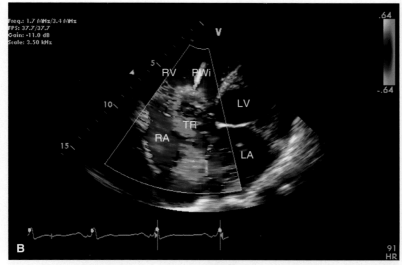

**Figure 14-5.** (*Continued*) **B:** Color Doppler shows severe TR suggestive of TV involvement and leaflet destruction.

## ABSCESS

- More commonly seen in left rather than right-sided endocarditis with a disposition for the **fibrous continuum** between the aortic and mitral annuli.
- **TEE is the test of choice to identify abscesses.** Sensitivity of TTE for abscess is <25%.
- There are no "typical" organisms that result in abscess.
- Rate of abscess with identified vegetation is 5% to 30%.
- Look for a **hypoechoic** area that may be **loculated** with surrounding thickened tissue that has heterogeneous echo-texture. **Assess the abscess for fistula formation using 2D and color Doppler** (Fig. 14-6).

## FISTULAS

- This should be considered particularly when a continuous murmur is heard in a patient with IE.
- Abscess at the right coronary sinus tends to fistulize to the RV and/or atrium (Fig. 14-7).
- Abscess near the non-coronary cusp tends to fistulize to the left atrium through the mitral-aortic fibrous continuum, which is relatively avascular compared to neighboring tissue.
- Fistulas may connect the aortic root with the left atrium.
- Best visualized with TEE given the usual involvement of the aortic annulus.
- Minimize the color Doppler window to maximize frame rate and look for flow.
- Check CW Doppler through the fistulous tract. Peak flow velocity should be consistent with the pressure difference between the aorta and the connecting chamber.

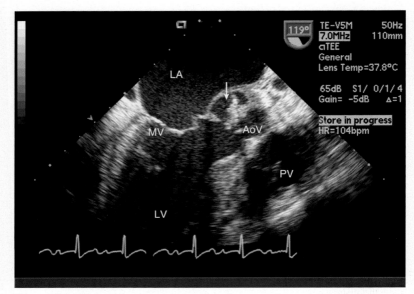

**Figure 14-6.** TEE 120 degree, LV long-axis view showing an abnormal septated cavity (*arrow*) in between the MV and AoV (fibrous continuum) extending to the aortic root consistent with aortic root abscess.

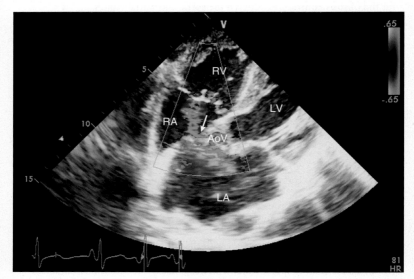

**Figure 14-7.** A5C with color Doppler shows high velocity jet originating from the right coronary sinus (*arrow*) and directed to the RA.

## PROSTHETIC VALVES

- Because of prosthetic-related artifact, patients suspected of IE with prosthetic valves should undergo TEE for further evaluation. This is especially true if multiple prosthetic valves are present (see Chapter 13).
- Sensitivity of TEE for prosthetic valve IE is 86% to 94% with a specificity of 88% to 99%.
- **Compared to native valves, in prosthetic valves the annulus instead of the leaflets is the more common initial site of infection.**
- Multiple components of the prosthesis need to be examined carefully.
- Sewing ring—check for a regular contour without an abnormal disruption. Both pannus and thrombus can disrupt the outline of the sewing ring in a similar fashion. Pannus tends to be echogenic/brighter compared to vegetations or thrombus.
- Bioprosthetic leaflets—examine the leaflets carefully for vegetations. Be aware that such leaflets can degenerate without any infectious etiology over the natural life of the valve. Such degeneration can look similar to that of damage secondary to infection. Regurgitation will be greater than the mild regurgitation that may be present with normal functioning valves.
- Mechanical leaflets—examination can be difficult secondary to artifact. Check the leaflets for symmetrical opening and closing angles. Examine whether a nonphysiologic gradient exists across the valve suggestive of obstruction.
- Valve apparatus—check for dehiscence of the valve apparatus from the myocardium that may cause a "rocking" motion of the valve if the dehiscence is large. The resulting perivalvular regurgitation is seen as an asymmetric turbulent jet on color Doppler (Fig. 14-8). Note that dehiscence can occur from infection and also disrupted sutures, friable myocardium, and excessive calcification. Finally, examine the perivalvular area for echolucent areas suggestive of abscess. Be aware that echo artifact from the valve may cause similar echolucency but will not be accompanied by a regurgitant jet.

---

- **Key Point:** *TEE is preferable for the evaluation of prosthetic valve or mechanical lead infection.*

---

## EMBOLIZATION

- Despite prompt recognition and treatment, embolization of vegetations remains a source of considerable morbidity and mortality.
- Risk of embolization reduces dramatically after the first 2 weeks of therapy.
- **Criteria associated with increased risk of embolization include right-sided endocarditis, vegetation length >10 mm, mitral valve involvement (particularly anterior leaflet), significantly mobile vegetations, and perivalvular extension.**

## INDICATIONS FOR SURGICAL CONSULTATION

- Congestive heart failure secondary to valvular insufficiency that is refractory to medical therapy
- Fungal IE (except *Histoplasma capsulatum*)
- Persistent sepsis (>72 hours) despite appropriate antibiotic therapy
- Valve dehiscence, rupture, abscess, or fistula

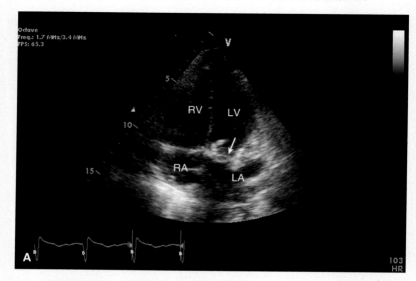

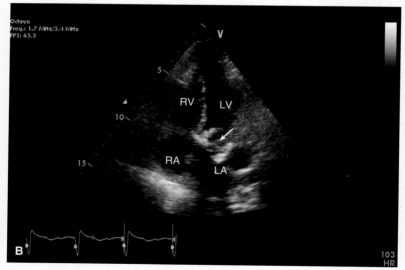

**Figure 14-8. A:** A4C with MV bioprosthesis (*arrow*) tilted toward the anterolateral wall in diastole. **B:** In systole the bioprosthesis tilts further and this movement back and forward throughout the cardiac cycle is called "rocking" suggestive of significant valve dehiscence.

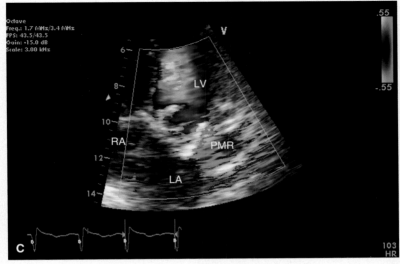

**Figure 14-8.** (*Continued*) **C:** Significant perivalvular mitral regurgitation (PMR) is seen on color Doppler.

- Anterior mitral leaflet infection in the setting of aortic valve IE
- Heart block caused by septal abscess
- Prosthetic valve endocarditis

## MONITORING OF INFECTIVE ENDOCARDITIS

- Diagnosis of IE made by TTE should be followed by TEE to assess for other valve involvement and complications that may not be visible by TTE.
- If the patient's clinical course deteriorates, TEE should be repeated.
- Following completion of therapy, TTE is preferred in order to establish a new baseline for comparison to future studies.

## FALSE POSITIVES FOR INFECTIVE ENDOCARDITIS

- Not all valvular vegetations are secondary to IE. Clinical correlation is necessary to assist in differentiating the following from IE:
  - Libman–Sacks endocarditis
  - Lambl's excrescences
  - Myxomatous valve disease
  - Myxoma
  - Papillary fibroelastoma
  - Acute rheumatic carditis
  - Prosthetic valve suture, pannus, or thrombus
  - Nodules of Arantius

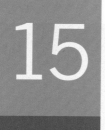

# 15 Pericardial Effusion and Cardiac Tamponade

Michael Yeung

## ANATOMY AND PHYSIOLOGY OF THE PERICARDIUM

- The pericardium consists of two layers: The **visceral pericardium**, which is adjacent to the epicardial surface of the heart and the **parietal pericardium**, which is a thicker, fibrous layer that encases most of the heart.
- The **pericardial space**, located in between these two layers, contains approximately 10 to 50 mL of pericardial fluid and allows the transmission of changes in intrathoracic pressure to the cardiac chambers. Therefore during inspiration; for example, both the intrathoracic pressure, pulmonary capillary wedge pressure (PCWP), and LV diastolic pressure fall in concert with minimal change in LV filling.
- The **pericardium** serves as a mechanical barrier between the heart and its adjacent mediastinal structures, a lubricant between the pericardial layers as well as a mechanical restraint on cardiac volume. This restraint is the reason why pressure and volume changes of one ventricle affect the other (**ventricular interdependence**).
- In the **normal respiratory cycle**, inspiration leads to a decrease in intrathoracic pressure, allowing for an increase in blood flow through the right side of the heart. Under normal conditions, the cardiac chambers and pericardium are compliant enough to accommodate for this increase in blood flow.
- In **tamponade ventricular interdependence is exaggerated** as transmission of changes in tamponade intrathoracic pressure to the ventricles and ventricular

compliance is diminished by an increase in intrapericardial pressure. During inspiration intrathoracic pressure decreases with a decrease in PCWP. LV diastolic pressure; however, does not decrease to the same degree because of increased intrapericardial pressure. This results in a reduction in LV filling pressure (PCWP-LV diastolic pressure) and is reflected in a reduced mitral E wave peak velocity. Increased venous return and reduced LV filling promotes increased RV filling reflected in an increased tricuspid E wave peak velocity. Reciprocal changes occur during expiration where LV filling is promoted to the detriment of RV filling.

- **Pulsus paradoxus** is a clinical manifestation of increased ventricular interdependence in tamponade, with a **decrease in systolic blood pressure >10 mmHg during inspiration.**
- The electrocardiographic sign of **electrical alternans** corresponds to the pendulum-like swinging of the heart within a large pericardial effusion now that the heart is not restrained by the pericardium.
- Once intrapericardial pressures exceed intracardiac pressures, chamber collapse is seen beginning with the lowest pressure chambers.

> - **Key Point:** *The **rate of accumulation** is just as important as the size of the pericardial effusion. A small but rapidly accumulating effusion may lead to tamponade with only 500 cc whereas a chronic effusion can accommodate up to 2000 cc of pericardial fluid before presenting with hemodynamic compromise.*

## ETIOLOGY OF PERICARDIAL DISEASE AND EFFUSIONS

- **Idiopathic**
- **Infectious**
  1. **Viral:** Echovirus, coxsackievirus, adenovirus, Hepatitis B, HIV
  2. **Bacterial:** Pneumococcus, Staphylococcus, Streptococcus, Mycobacterium
  3. **Fungal:** Histoplasmosis, coccidiomycosis
- **Immune/inflammatory**
  1. **Connective tissue disease:** SLE, Rheumatoid arthritis, Scleroderma
  2. **Postmyocardial infarction:** Dressler's syndrome
  3. **Uremic**
  4. **Postcardiac surgery**
  5. **Drug-induced:** Procainamide, hydralazine, isoniazid, cyclosporine
- **Neoplastic disease**
  1. **Direct extension:** Lung carcinoma, breast carcinoma
  2. **Metastatic:** Lymphoma, melanoma
  3. **Primary cardiac tumor**
- **Mechanical**
  1. **Blunt chest trauma**
  2. **Procedure related:** Percutaneous coronary intervention, implantation of pacemakers/defibrillators
  3. **Post-myocardial infarction free wall rupture**

## DIFFERENTIAL DIAGNOSIS OF ECHOLUCENT SPACE SURROUNDING THE HEART

- **Epicardial fat:** Usually presents as an isolated echolucent area anterior to the right ventricular free wall and spares the posterior pericardium. Epicardial fat can

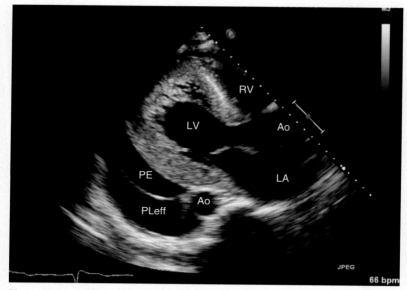

Figure 15-1. PLAX view of a pericardial effusion anterior to the descending aorta and a pleural effusion posterior to the aorta.

sometimes be identified as having a granular or specked appearance when compared to blood or pericardial fluid. Epicardial fat is more prevalent in the elderly, females, diabetics, patients with dyslipidemia and the obese.

• **Pleural effusion:** In the PLAX view, effusions seen anterior to the proximal descending thoracic aorta are pericardial whereas effusions that track posterior to the thoracic aorta are left-sided pleural effusions (Fig. 15-1). Left pleural effusions tend to localize primarily in the posterior–lateral aspect of the heart, while most pericardial effusions are present circumferentially unless it is loculated due to adhesions from surgery or an inflammatory process.

• **Simple pericardial effusion:** This tends to initially accumulate posteriorly in the oblique sinus. It is best seen in the PLAX view.

• **Loculated pericardial effusion:** Are often seen after cardiac surgery, mediastinal radiation or in long-standing inflammatory conditions that allows fibrin strands and adhesions to deposit along the pericardial space. This may lead to a localized increase in intrapericardial pressure with the absence of traditional echocardiographic signs of respiratory variation and diastolic collapse because of the absence of free-flowing fluid.

• **Key Point:** *Pericardial effusion and hematoma may be difficult to visualize immediately postcardiac surgery. Additional examination by transesophageal echocardiography should be considered if clinical suspicion for tamponade is high.*

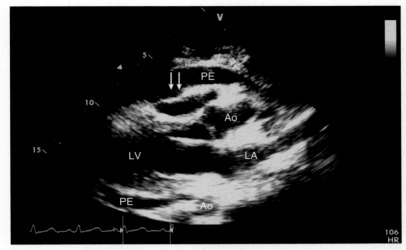

**Figure 15-2.** Simple concentric pericardial effusion in the PLAX view. Note diastolic compression of RV (*arrows*) suggestive of tamponade.

## ECHOCARDIOGRAPHIC ASSESSMENT OF CARDIAC TAMPONADE

### 2D Echocardiography

- **Pericardial effusion** is seen on 2D echocardiography as an echolucent space surrounding the heart (Fig. 15-2). A complex effusion is characterized by the presence of loculations, fibrinous strands, and thrombus (Fig. 15-3).
- The **size** of the pericardial effusion can be estimated in the PLAX, apical four-chamber (A4C), and subcostal views. Measurements are taken during end-diastole and the effusion is generally classified as:
  - Small if <0.5 cm from the LV wall
  - Moderate if between 0.5 to 2.0 cm from the LV wall
  - Large if >2 cm from the LV wall
- **Right atrial inversion** is best visualized in the A4C and subcostal views. Right atrial inversion begins to manifest when intrapericardial pressure is higher than the right atrium. This presents prior to the hemodynamic changes that lead to right ventricular diastolic collapse, given that RA pressure is lower than RV pressure. The duration of the inversion is important as well, and its presence for longer than one-third of the systolic period increases specificity for tamponade physiology (Fig. 15-4).
- **Right ventricular diastolic collapse** should be evaluated from multiple acoustic windows. M-mode shows a characteristic "dipping" of the anterior right ventricular free wall during diastole (Fig. 15-5). As in right atrial inversion, this occurs when intrapericardial pressure exceeds right ventricular pressure. This finding is more specific than right atrial systolic collapse for tamponade. The presence of RV diastolic collapse is correlated with a 20% decrease in cardiac output.

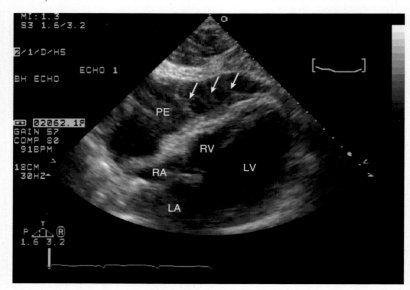

**Figure 15-3.** Complex pericardial effusion seen in the subcostal view with linear echodensities (*arrows*) attached along the compressed RA and RV free wall.

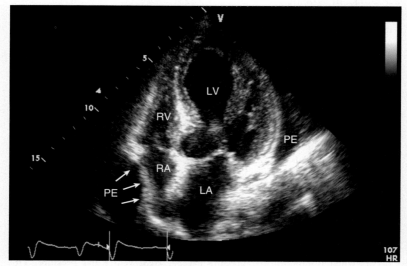

**Figure 15-4.** Marked right atrial collapse (*arrows*) in the apical four-chamber view.

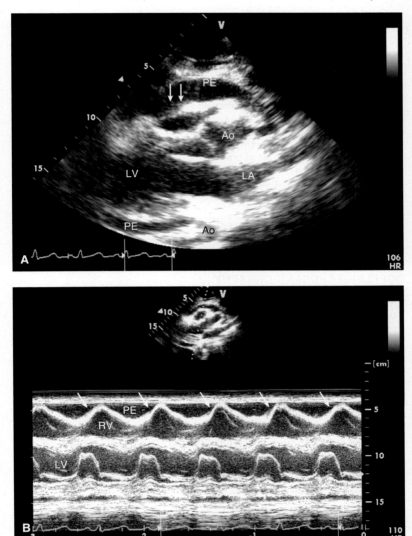

**Figure 15-5.** **(A)** Right ventricular diastolic collapse in the PLAX view with **(B)** corresponding M-mode image (*arrows*).

> • **Key Point:** *Patients with conditions that predispose them to elevated RV pressure or wall stiffness, as seen in pulmonary hypertension, infiltrative diseases, or atrial septal defects, will have a less pronounced or even absent RV diastolic collapse despite an elevated intrapericardial pressure.*

- **Paradoxical septal motion** highlights the physiology of respiratory variation and pulsus paradoxus and is best appreciated in the A4C view. During inspiration, the increased negative intracardiac pressure allows for greater filling of the RV. Given that the pericardial effusion, like a constricting elastic band around the heart, reduces compliance and expansion of the cardiac chambers, the septum shifts paradoxically toward the left ventricle during diastole—resulting in a lower stroke volume and lower systolic blood pressure during inspiration.
- In the subcostal view, visualization of a **dilated inferior vena cava** >2 cm with <50% collapse during inspiration as well as dilated hepatic veins suggests increased right atrial pressure lending support to elevated intracardiac pressures secondary to pericardial tamponade.

> • **Key Point:** *A fixed and dilated IVC may not be evident if the patient is undergoing mechanical ventilation or if the patient is hypovolemic.*

## DOPPLER ECHOCARDIOGRAPHY

- **Mitral and tricuspid respiratory variation:** In the A4C view, assessment of the mitral and tricuspid valve inflow velocities using PW Doppler at the leaflet tips is performed. At the respiratory physiology menu, **slow the sweep speed to 25 cm/s** to allow for an increased number of cardiac and respiratory cycles to be displayed. In tamponade, the increased blood flow entering the RV during inspiration corresponds to an increase tricuspid valve inflow velocity of approximately 40% or greater. Reciprocally, a decrease in mitral inflow velocity of approximately 25% or greater is seen.

> • **Key Point:** *Typically these changes occur on the **first beat** after the beginning of inspiration or expiration, differentiating tamponade from variation that occurs with diseases that result in large changes in intrathoracic pressures. For example, with severe obstructive airways disease, changes in mitral and tricuspid inflow occurs several beats after inspiration or expiration. Also, ensure that variation is not related to an irregular heart rhythm such as atrial fibrillation, which causes changes in the cardiac filling pattern unrelated to tamponade physiology (Fig. 15-6).*

## GENERAL CONSIDERATIONS

These echocardiographic signs are dependent on the balance between intrapericardial and intracardiac pressures. Patients with right ventricular hypertrophy or pulmonary hypertension for example may require higher intrapericardial pressures for two-dimensional and Doppler signs of tamponade to manifest.

Variation in mitral and tricuspid inflow is **volume** dependent and may not be present in patients with hypovolemia.

Most importantly cardiac tamponade is a **clinical diagnosis** and the echocardiographic signs described are only a "snap-shot" and guide to the clinical status of the patient.

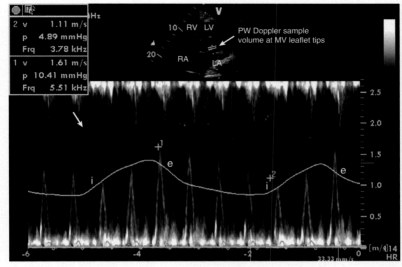

**Figure 15-6.** Pulsed-wave Doppler with sample volume at mitral leaflet tips recorded at a slow sweep speed. The green line indicates respirations with the beginning of inspiration (i) and expiration (e) labeled. Significant respiratory variation in the mitral valve Doppler inflow. Note timing of change in Doppler peak velocities compared to patient's respirations.

---

• **Key Point:** *Be aware that uncommonly, other pathology may mimic pericardial tamponade. For example, large pleural effusions or pneumothorax can compress the mediastinum increasing ventricular interdependence producing physiology similar to pericardial tamponade.*

---

## OTHER PERICARDIAL PATHOLOGY

Absent **congenital pericardium** occurs partially on the left side, while the complete absence of pericardium is extremely rare. Most patients are free of symptoms. Echocardiographically, this entity may manifest as exaggerated cardiac movement, abnormal ventricular septal motion, or partial displacement of cardiac structures to the left, giving the impression of right-sided enlargement and overload.

**Pericardial cysts** are typically benign and found incidentally. These cysts may be found predominantly by the left or right costophrenic angle. This is seen as a round, echo-free structure filled with fluid.

## EVALUATION OF CONSTRICTIVE PERICARDITIS

• Constrictive pericarditis should be considered in the evaluation of patients who present with heart failure despite normal left ventricular systolic function. This occurs due to a thickened and/or calcified pericardium which limits diastolic filling, leading to elevated filling pressures in the setting of normal contractile reserve.

> • **Key Point:** *In comparison to cardiac tamponade, where like a tight elastic band around the heart, increased pericardial pressure constantly affects LV filling and compliance, pericardial constriction is like encasing the heart in a small box that allows rapid expansion of the ventricles only to a point and then significantly limits further filling and markedly increases filling pressures.*

- Most common causes of constriction are prior cardiac surgery, mediastinal radiation, mediastinal infections, and collagen vascular diseases.
- Pericardial thickening and calcification typically have to be severe to be recognized on 2D echocardiographic images.
- Although nonspecific, **bi-atrial enlargement** representing elevated filling pressures, along with a normal systolic function may be indicative of constriction.
- Other features include rapid expansion and then sudden diastolic flattening of the left ventricular inferolateral wall ("heart in a box"), late diastolic interventricular septal bounce (septal movement reflects ventricular interdependence as the ventricles share a fixed pericardial volume—if one expands the other must shrink), IVC dilatation, increased hepatic Doppler flow reversal during **expiration** and significant atrio-ventricular valve inflow respiratory variation in the **absence of a pericardial effusion** (Fig. 15-7). More subtle findings of increased intracardiac filling pressures such as premature opening of the pulmonic valve may also be present.
- Pulmonary pressures are often normal in patients with constrictive pericarditis, as opposed to restrictive cardiomyopathy where pulmonary pressures >60 mmHg is commonly seen.
- **"Annulus paradoxus"** refers to the phenomenon where in constrictive pericarditis despite increased filling pressures, the mitral septal annular velocity is normal (≥8 cm/s) as opposed to myocardial or infiltrative diseases when it is reduced. This is based on the fact that in constriction, alterations in ventricular filling are related to an abnormal, less compliant pericardium with the **myocardium being normal**. This is in contrast to infiltrative disease where ventricular filling is impaired secondary to abnormal myocardial relaxation, reflected in reducing annular velocities as the disease progresses.

> • **Key Point:** *In contrast to normal hearts, in constrictive pericarditis, the mitral septal annular velocity (e') may be higher than the lateral annulus secondary to (1) tethering of the lateral wall from the adjacent thickened, adherent pericardium and (2) exaggerated motion of the unencumbered septal wall ("annulus reversus") (Fig. 15-8).*

## DIFFERENTIATION OF CONSTRICTIVE PERICARDITIS AND RESTRICTIVE CARDIOMYOPATHY

- Adjunct modalities such as cardiac catheterization, computed tomography, or magnetic resonance imaging may be needed to aid in the differentiation of constrictive pericarditis from restrictive cardiomyopathy.
- Left ventricular myocardial thickness is often increased in restrictive cardiomyopathy in contrast to constrictive disease where in contrast the pericardium is abnormally thickened or calcified.
- Both conditions exhibit elevated left and right atrial filling pressures.
- Pulmonary artery systolic pressures are elevated in restrictive cardiomyopathy (>60 mmHg) whereas this is often normal in constrictive pericarditis unless there is an underlying primary pulmonary pathology.

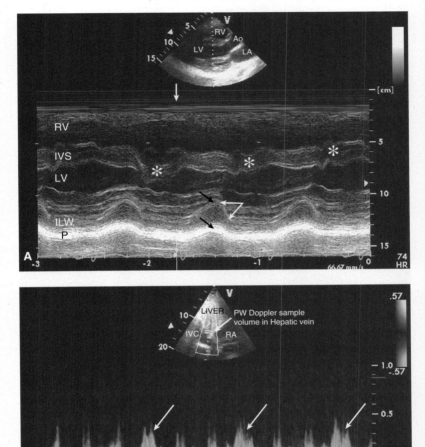

**Figure 15-7.** Patient with constrictive pericarditis. **(A)** PLAX M-mode at the base of the ventricles shows exaggerated inferolateral wall motion with rapid and abrupt cessation of motion during diastole without further expansion (*double headed arrow*). "Tracking" of the pericardium with the inferior–lateral wall is seen suggesting attachment (*short black arrows*). Inter-ventricular late diastolic dip back toward the LV is seen (*). **(B)** Hepatic Doppler shows increased flow reversals (*long arrows*) during expiration (e).

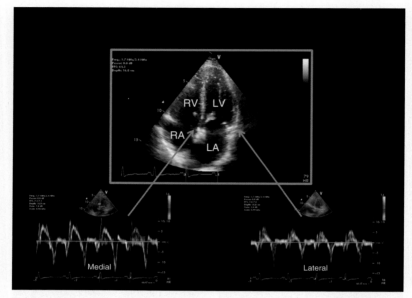

**Figure 15-8.** Patient with constrictive pericarditis with "annulus paradoxus". The mitral annular peak early velocity is greater than the lateral annulus (reverse of normal). This is because of adherent pericardium reducing lateral motion and compensatory exaggerated septal motion.

- Because ventricular compliance is impaired, the diastolic filling pattern is similar in both constrictive pericarditis and advanced restrictive cardiomyopathy.
- A feature of both entities is that both conditions display diastolic flow reversal of the hepatic vein Doppler. But whereas the hepatic vein flow reversal is more prominent during **inspiration** for the restrictive cardiomyopathies ("sick RV" cannot accommodate increased venous return), the diastolic flow reversal is increased during **expiration** for constrictive pericarditis (RV volume is limited by expansion of the LV—ventricular interdependence).
- Left ventricular strain analysis can also be applied to differentiate both conditions. A reduced circumferential strain and early diastolic apical untwisting velocities is consistent with pericardial constriction (**outer fibers** involved in these movements). In contrast, restrictive cardiomyopathy displays a reduced longitudinal displacement and e′ (subendocardial fibers involved in these movements).

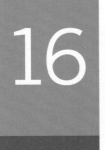

# 16 Diseases of the Great Vessels: Aorta and Pulmonary Artery

Anupama Rao

**HIGH-YIELD FINDINGS: AORTA AND PULMONARY ARTERY**

- Aortic root measurements are made in a modified parasternal long-axis view at end-diastole.
- It is important to index aortic size for body surface area. Indications for surgical correction are based on the underlying condition.
- With aortic dissection, determine where flow in systole is occurring—this usually identifies the true lumen.
- Intramural hematomas are treated similarly to aortic dissection.
- McConnell's sign in combination with 60/60 sign is specific for pulmonary emboli.

**KEY TTE VIEWS: AORTA AND PULMONARY ARTERY**

- Standard parasternal long axis: Descending aorta in cross-section
- Modified parasternal long axis (probe is placed in a superior rib space than standard PLAX): Aortic valve annulus, sinuses of Valsalva, sinotubular junction, ascending aorta
- Right ventricular outflow view: Main pulmonary artery
- PSAX: Aortic valve leaflets, sinuses of Valsalva, right ventricular outflow tract, and main pulmonary artery
- Off-axis A4C and A2C (posterior tilt): Descending aorta
- Subcostal view (long axis): Proximal abdominal aorta
- Suprasternal notch: Aortic arch, identification of branch vessels: Inominate, carotid and subclavian arteries, descending aorta, right pulmonary artery

While transthoracic echocardiography (TTE) provides useful serial measurement of the great vessels, transesophageal echocardiography (TEE) is the ultrasound modality of choice in comprehensively imaging these structures, especially in emergency situations.

## AORTA

### Anatomy

- The aorta is divided into the thoracic and abdominal aorta.
- The thoracic aorta is further divided into the aortic root, arch and ascending and descending aorta.

- The aortic root consists of the aortic annulus, the sinuses of Valsalva and the sino-tubular junction, which joins the proximal ascending portion of the thoracic aorta (Fig. 16-1).
- The ascending portion continues until the origin of the inominate artery.
- The aortic arch gives rise to the inominate, left main carotid, and left subclavian arteries.
- The descending aorta begins after the origin of the left subclavian artery and continues past the diaphragm becoming the abdominal aorta (Fig. 16-2). The ligamentum arteriosum is just distal to the left subclavian artery, anchoring the descending aorta to the thorax.

> • **Key Point:** *This area in between the ligamentum arteriosum and the left subclavian artery is known as the **aortic isthmus**, which is the most common location for abnormalities such as coarctation, patent ductus arteriosus, and dissection due to trauma or deceleration injury.*

TEE is an excellent modality to image the entire aorta apart from a small "blind-spot" where the air-filled trachea shields a segment of the distal ascending aorta as it becomes the proximal aortic arch.

## Key TEE Views

- Upper esophageal (20 to 25 cm) 0-degree long axis: Aortic arch
- Upper esophageal (20 to 25 cm) 90-degree short axis: Aortic arch along with pulmonary artery
- Mid-esophageal (30 to 40 cm) 30- to 40-degree short axis: Aortic valve
- Mid-esophageal (30 to 40 cm) 100- to 120-degree left ventricular long-axis view: Aortic valve and root
- Deep transgastric view (45 to 50 cm) 0- to 20-degree flexion: Aortic valve and root
- Turning probe posteriorly: Transgastric to upper esophageal views 0- and 90-degree views of thoracic aorta

## Pathology

### Aortic Aneurysm

An aortic aneurysm is defined as the presence of dilatation of over 50% of the normal diameter (>2.75 cm/m$^2$), involving all three layers of the vessel (intima, media, and adventitia). Etiologies include hypertension, atherosclerosis, poststenotic dilation, cystic medial necrosis, collagen vascular diseases such as Marfan's syndrome and systemic lupus erythematosus as well as inflammatory states such as rheumatoid arthritis and Reiter's syndrome.

> • **Key Point:** *Patients with Marfan's syndrome usually have a pattern of aortic dilatation, which starts in the sinuses of Valsalva and expands distally ("pear"-shaped aortic root) (Fig. 16-3).*

Measurements of aortic diameter are usually made in the modified parasternal long-axis view at end-diastole. Serial annual echocardiographic measurements are made once aortic dilatation (upper normal limit is 2.1 cm/m$^2$ at aortic sinuses) is detected.

Measurements include:

- Aortic annulus
- Sinuses of Valsalva

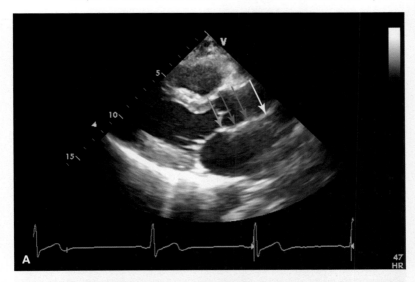

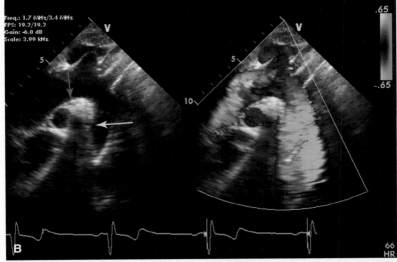

**Figure 16-1.** **(A)** PLAX (blue, aortic annulus; red, sinuses of Valsalva; green, sinotubular junction; white, proximal ascending aorta) and **(B)** suprasternal notch (SSN) views demonstrating measurements for the aortic root and arch respectively (cyan, aortic arch; yellow, descending aorta).

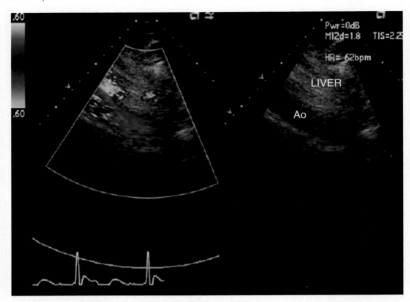

Figure 16-2. Subcostal view of the abdominal aorta.

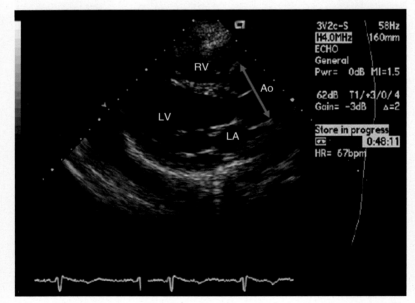

Figure 16-3. PLAX view showing aortic root dilatation at the sinuses of Valsalva (*double-headed arrow*) in a patient with Marfan's syndrome.

- Sinotubular junction
- Proximal ascending aorta
- Aortic arch (suprasternal view)
- Abdominal aorta (subcostal view)

*Indications for Operative Intervention for Thoracic Aneurysms*
- Ascending aorta or aortic sinus diameter ≥5.5 cm
- Genetically mediated disorders with higher risk of dissection (e.g., Marfans, Ehlers Danlos, Bicuspid aortic valve, Turner's syndrome, Loeys–Dietz syndrome, Familial thoracic aortic aneurysm or dissection) ≥4–5 cm depending on condition
- Ascending aorta or aortic root >4.5 cm in patients already undergoing aortic valve replacement
- Rapidly expanding aneurysms (>5 mm/year) when ascending aorta or aortic sinus <5.5 cm

*Sinus of Valsalva Aneurysm*
- These aneurysms usually involve abnormal dilatation of one of the sinuses of Valsalva (Fig. 16-4).
- Sinus of Valsalva aneurysms (SVA) may be congenital or due to processes that involve the aortic root such as Marfan's syndrome, syphilis, endocarditis, trauma, or prior surgery.
- SVA may appear as a "windsock" deformity projecting into adjacent structures.
- SVAs originate most commonly from the **right coronary sinus**.

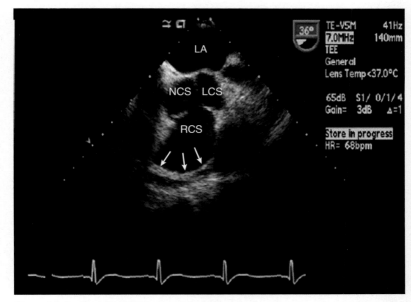

**Figure 16-4.** Short-axis TEE image of the aortic valve demonstrating a large right coronary sinus of Valsalva aneurysm (NCS, non-coronary sinus; LCS, left coronary sinus; RCS, right coronary sinus).

- Aneurysms of the right coronary sinus protrude into the RV outflow tract, while left coronary sinus aneurysms protrude into the left atrium and the non-coronary sinus into the right atrium.

  - **Key Point:** *Rupture of SVA into adjacent structures is the main cause of mortality. Cardiac tamponade can occur if rupture occurs into the pericardial sac.*

- Associated conditions include ventricular septal defect (VSD), bicuspid aortic valve, aortic regurgitation, pulmonary stenosis, atrial septal defect (ASD), and coarctation of the aorta.

### Aortic Dissection

- 2D echocardiography is routinely performed in emergency situations to rapidly diagnose aortic dissection. This is usually a catastrophic event triggered by a tear in the aortic intima, which subsequently leads to dissection within the underlying media and creation of a false lumen.
- Most dissections occur in the ascending aorta just distal to the aortic valve and in the descending portion distal to the left subclavian artery.
- Factors which predispose patients to dissection, include hypertension, bicuspid aortic valve, cystic medial necrosis, trauma, pregnancy, cocaine use, connective tissue disease, prolonged steroid use, inflammatory arteritis such as giant cell arteritis and iatrogenic trauma.
- Two main classification systems have been used to describe aortic dissections, namely the Stanford and Debakey systems.
- In the Debakey classification, Type I originates in the ascending aorta propagating to the arch. It may involve other sections of the aorta as well, Type II is limited to the ascending aorta only and Type III involves the descending aorta only.
- With the Stanford system, Type A is any dissection involving the ascending aorta (including Debakey Type I and Type II) and Type B only involves the descending aorta (Debakey Type III).

  - **Key Point:** *Dissections involving the ascending aorta require prompt surgical management while those which involve only the descending portion may respond better to medical therapy.*

## 2D and Doppler Findings

- Dilated aortic root.
- Linear mobile echodensity representing an intimal flap (high specificity for dissection)
- Differential color Doppler in false and true lumens; the true lumen usually fills with blood during systole, while the false lumen has variable flow (Fig. 16-5). Entry points between the two lumens may be seen as areas of turbulence on color Doppler. Occasionally swirling, low velocity flow may be noted in the false lumen with areas of partial or complete thrombosis.

  - **Key Point:** *Although it is sometimes difficult to distinguish the true lumen from the false lumen, the false lumen is usually larger than the true lumen in diastole with the true lumen expanding during systole.*

- Complications of aortic dissection include pericardial effusion, tamponade, aortic regurgitation (aortic root dilatation or flail aortic valve leaflet secondary to dissection flap), wall motion abnormalities caused by dissection extending into coronary artery

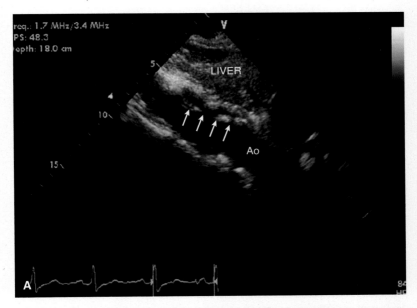

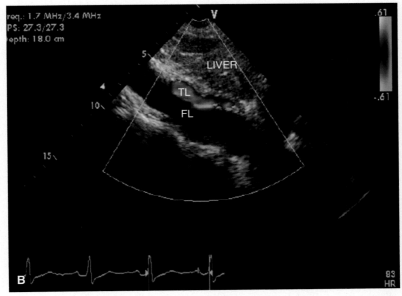

**Figure 16-5. (A)** Subcostal view demonstrating a dissection flap (*arrows*) in the abdominal aorta with **(B)** flow seen in the true lumen on color Doppler (TL, true lumen; FL, false lumen).

• M-mode can demonstrate dissociation between movement of the intimal flap and the wall of the aorta

> • **Key Point:** *The intimal flap usually moves toward the false lumen in systole.*

Given that the esophagus lies in close proximity to the thoracic aorta the higher spatial resolution of TEE has a very high sensitivity and specificity (99% and 98%) for the diagnosis of aortic dissection (Figs. 16-6 and 16-7).

> • **Key Point:** *In the suprasternal view, at times, the inominate vein can be mistaken for a dissection flap. Color Doppler of the area can be used to distinguish vein from a dissection flap. It is important to recognize this as a **normal** anatomic finding (Fig. 16-8).*

### Intramural Hematoma

• Intramural hematoma is characterized by heterogeneous thickening of the aortic wall **>7 mm in a crescentic or circular pattern** (Fig. 16-9).
• This usually involves rupture of the vasa-vasorum into the media and intramural blood and thrombus may be present.
• This can be differentiated from dissection, as there is no intimal flap or blood flow within the thickened wall.

> • **Key Point:** *About a third of intramural hematomas progress to overt aortic dissection or rupture and hence are clinically treated similarly to dissection.*

### Coarctation of Aorta

This is a congenital condition involving narrowing of the descending aorta at the site of the ligamentum arteriosum, immediately distal to the left subclavian artery. Associated conditions include Turner's syndrome, bicuspid aortic valve, patent ductus arteriosus, VSD, and intracranial aneurysms. There are three types of coarctation:

• Preductal: Narrowing proximal to ductus arteriosus
• Ductal: Narrowing at insertion of ductus arteriosus
• Postductal: Narrowing distal to ductus arteriosus

Coarctation of the aorta is best seen in the suprasternal view by TTE and in high esophageal views by TEE.

## 2D Findings

• Suprasternal view: Tapering or discrete area of narrowing of the proximal descending aorta (Fig. 16-10)
• Poststenotic dilatation may be present
• Left ventricular hypertrophy

## CW and PW Doppler

• Increased velocity across coarctation in descending aorta (Fig. 16-11)
• Estimate peak gradient across coarctation with modified Bernoulli equation: $\Delta P = 4 \times v^2$
• "Shark-tooth" pattern describes a systolic peak with slowly decremental diastolic flow related to distal diastolic run-off if significant collateral circulation is present

> • **Key Point:** *Be aware of different Doppler patterns in the suprasternal notch view (Fig. 16-12).*

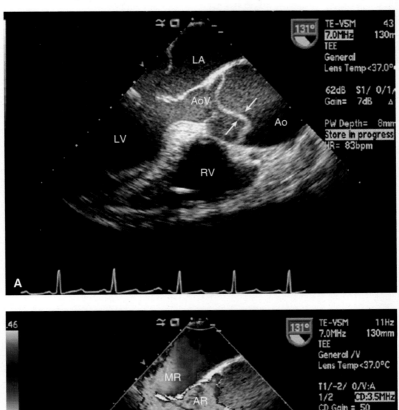

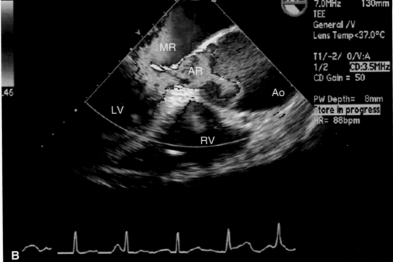

Figure 16-6. A: TEE LV long-axis image demonstrating a dissection flap (*arrows*) in the aortic root causing a flail noncoronary cusp of the aortic valve. B: Severe aortic regurgitation is seen as well as *diastolic* mitral regurgitation secondary to elevated LV end-diastolic pressure.

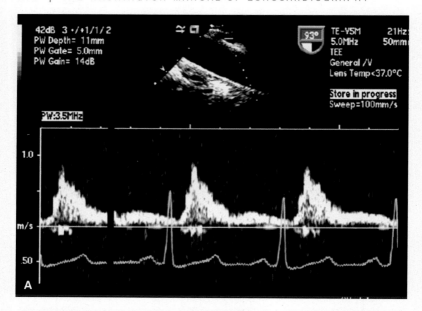

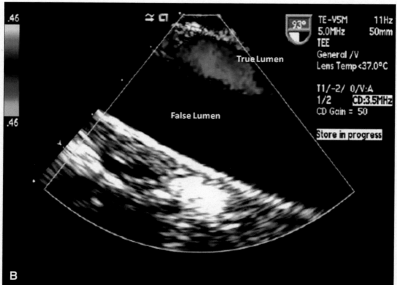

**Figure 16-7. A:** TEE image of a descending thoracic aorta dissection at 90 degrees, with color Doppler demonstrating flow in the true lumen. **B:** Pulsed-wave Doppler confirms systolic flow in the true lumen.

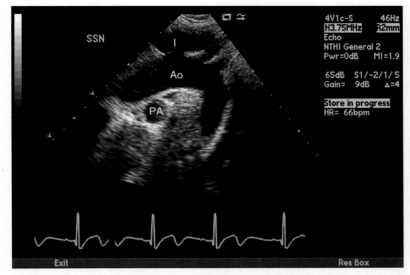

**Figure 16-8.** Inominate vein seen adjacent to the aortic arch in the suprasternal notch view.

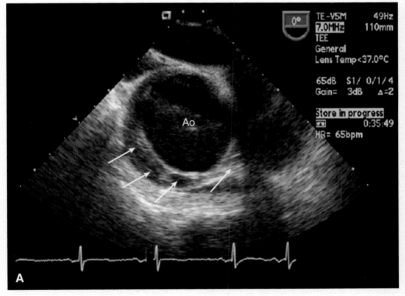

**Figure 16-9. A:** TEE short-axis image of the descending thoracic aorta showing the classic crescentic shape of an intramural hematoma (*arrows*).(*continued*)

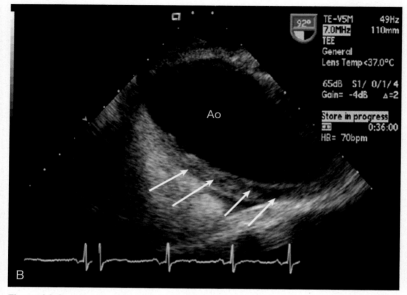

**Figure 16-9.** (*Continued*) **B:** This is also seen on the corresponding 90-degree view.

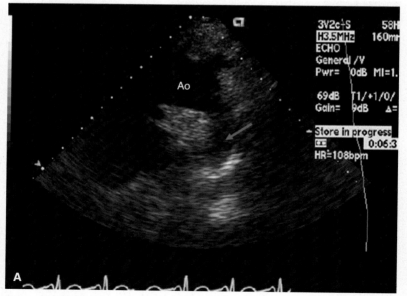

**Figure 16-10. A:** Suprasternal notch view of the aortic arch with a marked reduction in caliber of the lumen see at the proximal descending aorta (*arrow*).

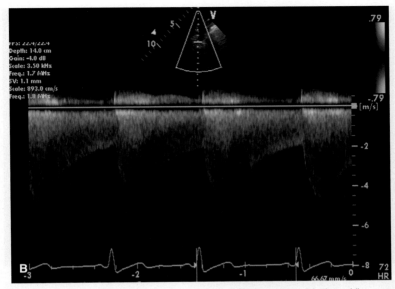

**Figure 16-10.** (*Continued*) **B:** CW Doppler demonstrates the classic "shark-tooth" pattern associated with aortic coarctation. There is an early elevated peak velocity followed by a slow taper of the Doppler envelope related to diastolic "run-off" in the collateral circulation.

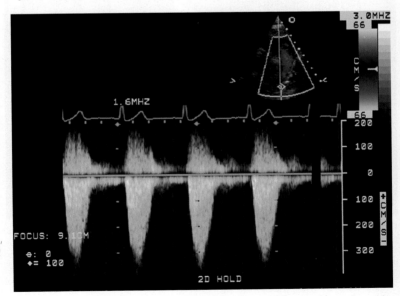

**Figure 16-11.** CW Doppler in the suprasternal notch view of the aorta in a patient with a history of *coarctation repair*. Note the high peak velocities seen in the descending without diastolic "run-off" related to residual narrowing of the aorta.

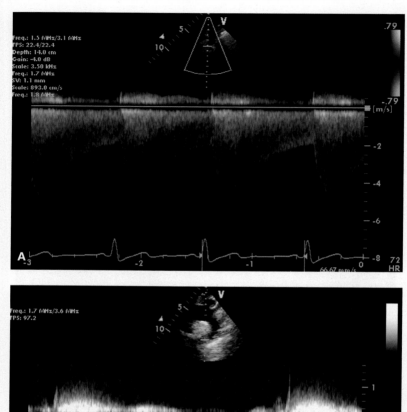

**Figure 16-12.** Comparison of abnormal Doppler patterns acquired from the suprasternal notch view. **(A)** CW Doppler of the descending aorta demonstrating the classic pattern of aortic coarctation. **(B)** CW Doppler detecting an elevated systolic velocity secondary to right pulmonary artery stenosis.

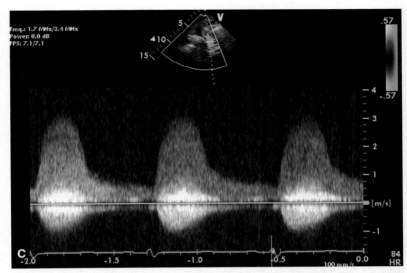

Figure 16-12. (*Continued*) (**C**) CW Doppler detecting an elevated systolic velocity (note, toward the probe) secondary to significant stenosis of the left subclavian artery.

*Aortic Atherosclerosis*

Aortic atherosclerosis is a known risk factor for ischemic stroke, peripheral embolic events and is correlated with coronary artery disease. TEE is an excellent imaging modality to identify aortic atherosclerotic plaque as it allows for detailed visualization of the entire thoracic aorta (Fig. 16-13).

- **Key Point:** *Atheromas that measure >5 mm, are mobile, pedunculated or protruding and those with an irregular intimal surface have been demonstrated to be more likely to result in embolic events.*

## PULMONARY ARTERY

### Anatomy

The main pulmonary artery begins at the base of the right ventricle and gives rise to right and left main stem branches, which deliver deoxygenated blood to the lungs.

### Key Views

- PLAX right ventricular outflow view: Main pulmonary artery
- PSAX at the level of the aortic valve: Right ventricular outflow tract, main pulmonary artery, and bifurcation (Fig. 16-14)
- Suprasternal view: Right pulmonary artery visualized in cross section posterior to ascending aorta and beneath aortic arch

### Pathology

*Pulmonary Artery Dilatation*

Dilatation of the pulmonary artery can be found in conjunction with a number of conditions including right-sided volume overload, pulmonary hypertension

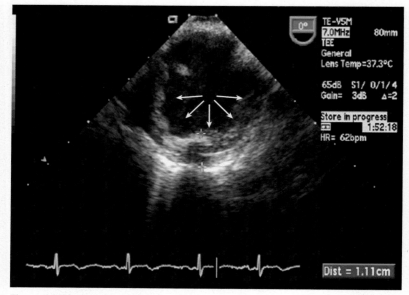

**Figure 16-13.** TEE short-axis view of the descending thoracic aorta demonstrating severe aortic atherosclerosis (*arrows*).

(Fig. 16-15), congenital pulmonary artery stenosis, transposition of great vessels and is rarely idiopathic.

*Pulmonary Embolism*

While TTE is not recommended as a routine test to confirm pulmonary embolism (PE) there are useful signs to suggest this diagnosis and findings important for risk stratification and management. Acute PE can affect right-sided heart function due to a sudden increase in pulmonary arterial resistance. Echocardiographic findings of right heart strain have been well documented to carry a worse prognosis and may indicate a need for more aggressive measures such as thrombectomy or intravenous thrombolytic therapy.

## 2D and Doppler Findings of PE

- Free floating thrombus in RV or "clot in transit"—very rare, but diagnostic of PE (main PA/saddle embolism) (Fig. 16-16)
- PLAX right ventricular end-diastolic dimension/left ventricular end-diastolic dimension ratio >0.7
- Right ventricular enlargement, free wall hypokinesis
  - Abrupt rise in pulmonary artery pressure
  - McConnell sign: Normal to hyperdynamic motion of the right ventricle apex, with akinesis of the right ventricle mid free wall; high specificity for PE (Fig. 16-17)
  - Interventricular paradoxic septal movement; "D-shaped" septum in parasternal short axis suggestive of pulmonary hypertension; Often, LV cavity is small in size (Fig. 16-18)
- 60/60 sign: Right ventricle systolic pressure <60 mmHg + RVOT acceleration time <60 ms (Fig. 16-19)

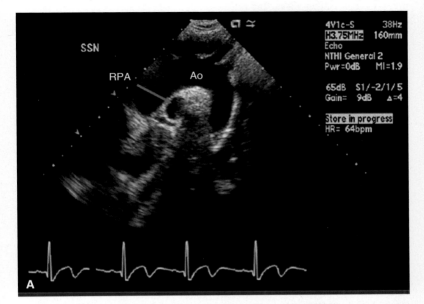

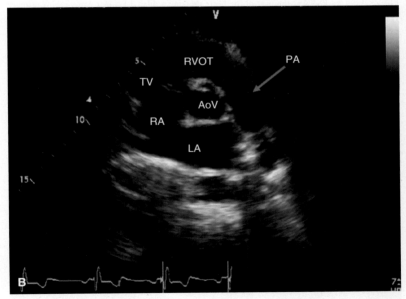

**Figure 16-14. A:** Suprasternal notch view with the right pulmonary artery (RPA) seen underneath aortic arch. **B:** PSAX view at the aortic level showing the main pulmonary artery (PA) (*arrow*) prior to bifurcation.

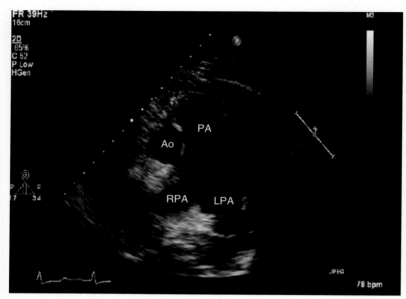

**Figure 16-15.** PSAX at the base of the heart showing a dilated PA in a patient with primary pulmonary hypertension (RPA, right pulmonary artery; LPA, left pulmonary artery).

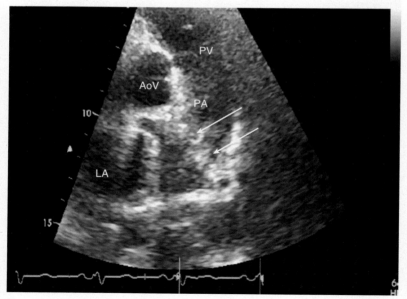

**Figure 16-16.** PSAX at the base of the heart with a saddle embolism (*arrows*) seen in the PA.

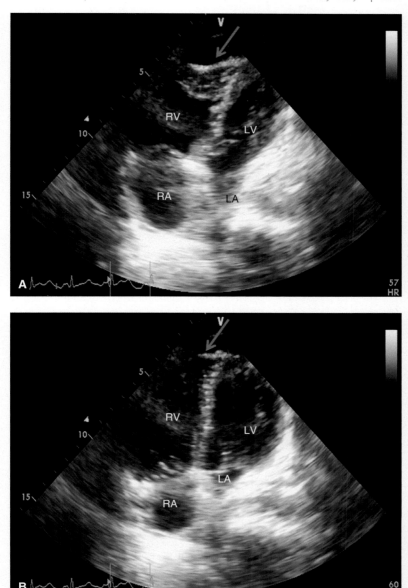

**Figure 16-17.** A4C view in (**A**) systole and (**B**) diastole showing right ventricular enlargement and McConnell's sign with apical hyperkinesis (*arrow*) and RV basal to mid free wall hypokinesis in a patient with a pulmonary embolism.

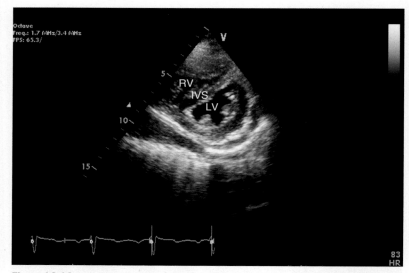

**Figure 16-18.** PSAX at the papillary muscle level demonstrating enlarged RV and "D-shaped" LV with interventricular septal flattening in a patient with severe pulmonary hypertension.

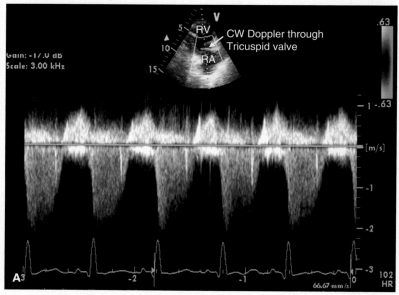

**Figure 16-19.** "60/60" sign in patient with acute pulmonary embolism. **(A)** CW Doppler through the tricuspid valve demonstrates a peak tricuspid regurgitant gradient <60 mmHg.

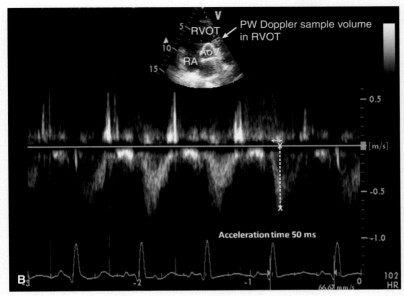

**Figure 16-19.** (*Continued*) **(B)** PSAX PW Doppler in the RVOT shows an acceleration time (*double-headed arrow*) <60 ms.

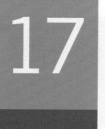

# 17 Congenital Heart Disease

Thomas K. Kurian, Mohammed K. Saghir, and Daniel H. Cooper

In recognizing the complexity of this topic, this chapter is intended to give an introduction to congenital abnormalities that may be seen in the adult population. Many of the patients will already have had some form of palliative or corrective surgery. In this regard, it is critical to obtain a thorough history of prior evaluation and treatment, as this will significantly impact the focus of image acquisition and interpretation.

Basic echocardiographic approach for evaluating unknown congenital heart disease (adapted from Diagnosis and Management of Adult Congenital Heart Disease by Gatzoulis):

- *Establish apex position:* Using a standard subcostal view (probe indicator points to patient's left shoulder) if the apex of the heart is pointing to the right of the patient's body = dextrocardia, to the left = levocardia (normal!).
- *Establish situs of atria:* Using a standard subcostal view of the aorta and IVC in cross section with color Doppler (probe perpendicular to spine with indicator pointing to the patient's left hip), determine whether the aorta (red) is to the left and IVC (blue) to the right (situs solitus-normal!) or opposite (situs inversus) of the spine (Fig. 17-1). Atrial situs follows abdominal situs in ~80% of patients.
- *Identify the morphologic RV:* Trabeculated, moderator band present, apically displaced TV compared to MV, septal attachment of TV.
- *Establish the great vessels:* PA early branching, aortic root gives off coronary arteries.

---

- **Key Point:** *AV valves always stay with their respective ventricle, that is the apically displaced TV establishes its ventricle as the morphologic RV.*

---

## I. SIMPLE SHUNTS

### KEY CONCEPTS

- L→R shunt allows a portion of the pulmonary venous return to escape back to the lungs and reduces the cardiac output by the amount of the shunted volume.
- R→L shunt: Oxygen content of systemic arterial blood falls in proportion to the volume of de-oxygenated systemic venous blood that has bypassed the lungs mixing with normal pulmonary venous return
- To calculate shunt fraction (pulmonary flow/systemic flow = Qp/Qs) measure area of both LVOT and RVOT, trace PW Doppler through each valve to get VTI.

$$Qp/Qs = CSA_{RVOT} \times VTI_{RVOT}/CSA_{LVOT} \times VTI_{LVOT}$$

- Qp/Qs >1 : 1 indicates pulmonary flow exceed systemic flow and defines a net L→R shunt as volume of shunted oxygenated blood + venous blood entering the pulmonary circuit exceeds amount of blood leaving the systemic circuit.

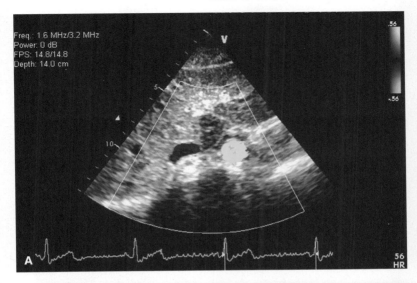

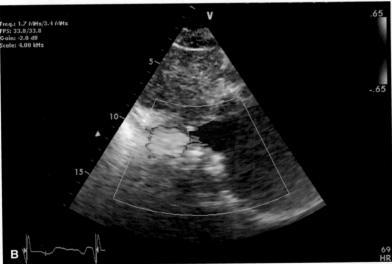

Figure 17-1. Subcostal cross-sectional view with color Doppler to establish atrial situs. A: IVC (blue) to the right and abdominal aorta (yellow) to the right in situs solitus (normal!). B: IVC to the left and abdominal aorta to the right in a patient with situs inversus.

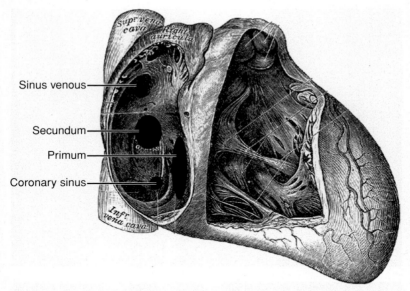

Sinus venous

Secundum

Primum

Coronary sinus

**Figure 17-2.** Anatomic distribution of ASD as seen from the right atrium. (Adapted from Gray, H. *Anatomy of the Human Body*, 20th ed. Philadelphia: Lea & Febiger, 1918.)

- Qp/Qs <1:1 indicates net R→L shunt as venous de-oxygenated blood mixes with oxygenated systemic blood.
- **Qp/Qs >1.5:1 is considered a significant L→R shunt *especially if right heart chamber dilatation is present.***

A. **ASD**

See Figure 17-2.

**Types:**
- *Secundum:* 75% of ASDs; located near the foramen ovale (mid interatrial septum).
- *Primum:* 15% of ASDs; associated with AV canal defects (AVCD; base of interatrial septum).
- *Sinus venosus:* 10% of ASDs; posterior edge of interatrial septum; usually associated with partial anomalous pulmonary venous return (typically right superior pulmonary vein).
- *Coronary sinus ASD:* Rare; absence of the common wall that separates the LA from the coronary sinus as it courses in the AV groove to the RA. It is associated with persistent left superior vena cava.

**Hemodynamics**
- Flow across an ASD is determined by the difference in compliance and capacity of both ventricles.
- The thick walled LV is less compliant and under higher pressure than the thin walled RV and this favors L→R shunting.
- Pulmonary blood flow is subsequently increased over time leading to **RV volume overload** (dilated RV, diastolic flattening of interventricular septum).

- The right heart tolerates volume overload much better than pressure overload and therefore symptoms develop late, once pulmonary vascular resistance and pressures eventually increase.
- Eisenmenger's syndrome occurs when right heart pressures exceed left heart pressures promoting R→L shunt and hypoxemia.

---

- **Key Point:** *Best views to locate ASD are the PSAX, A4C, and subcostal. Beware of "drop-out" of the interatrial septum in the A4C view related to reduced lateral resolution of the ultrasound beam that may mimic a secundum ASD. This should be confirmed in the subcostal view where the interatrial septum is perpendicular to the ultrasound beam and also by color and pulsed-wave Doppler. Typically ASD flow begins in systole and continues throughout the cardiac cycle with **a broad peak in late systole and early diastole** (Fig. 17-3).*

---

- **Key Point:** *The subcostal and "off-axis" subcostal views are typically the only views in which a sinus venosus ASD may be visualized (Fig. 17-4). A TEE should be performed to assess for sinus venosus ASD in patients with unexplained right heart volume overload, especially if the agitated saline study is markedly positive without a shunt location identified.*

---

### Surgical repair
- ASD closed if there is evidence of right ventricular dilatation or ASD diameter ≥10 mm
- Surgical repair or trans-catheter closure

### Echocardiography
- TTE and TEE should document the type and size of ASD (ASD diameter) as well as direction (color and spectral Doppler), significance of shunt (QP/QS) and presence of associated congenital lesions.
- Post trans-catheter closure assess for maintenance of position of the occluder and any residual shunt (Fig. 17-5). Usually a small residual shunt is noted immediately after occluder placement, which should eventually cease.

---

- **Key Point:** *Injection of agitated saline results in a **quick** (<3 to 4 beats), **intense** opacification of the LV **that clears** with subsequent beats.*

---

- Identify AV valve defects—for example, cleft MV in patients with ostium primum ASD.

## B. VSD
See Figure 17-6.

### Types:
- *Perimembranous:* 80% of VSDs, located near the septal leaflet of the TV and below the aortic valve.
- *Muscular:* Either single or multiple ("Swiss-cheese" septum) involving the septum (Fig. 17-7).
- *Inlet:* Involves the inflow portion of the septum and is associated with AVCD.
- *Supracristal or outflow tract:* Involves RV outflow tract (above crista supraventricularis) and near the outflow valves; frequently occluded by a cusp of the aortic valve causing AR.

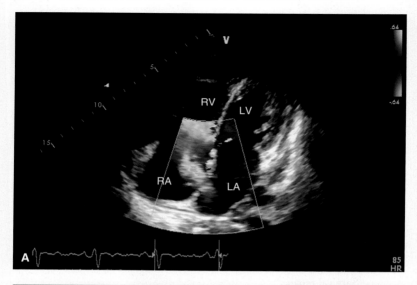

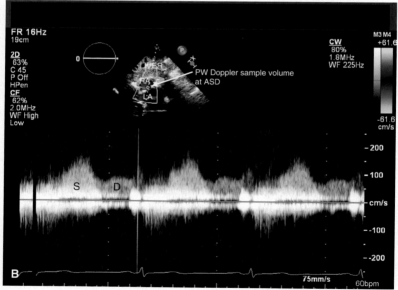

**Figure 17-3. A:** A4C with color Doppler demonstrating L → R flow across a secundum ASD. **B:** Pulsed-wave Doppler across the secundum ASD in a subcostal view demonstrating the characteristic broad peak flow in late systole and early diastole.

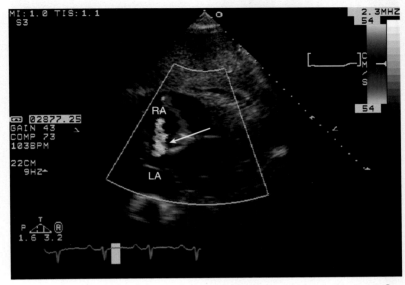

**Figure 17-4.** An off-axis subcostal image with color Doppler demonstrating L→R flow (*arrow*) at the posterior aspect of the interatrial septum consistent with a sinus venosus ASD.

### Hemodynamics

- The majority of small single VSDs close spontaneously in childhood. A minority will persist into adulthood requiring surgical intervention.
- The majority of flow occurs in **systole** resulting in an unmistakable, loud pansystolic murmur.
- The shunt is initially L→R increasing flow to the pulmonary circulation and back to the LV.
- Pulmonary artery systolic pressure (PASP) can be estimated, in the absence of pulmonic stenosis or RV outflow tract obstruction, if the systolic blood pressure (SBP) is known (PASP = SBP − $4V_{VSD}^2$).
- "Restrictive" VSDs are small high velocity/gradient jets (typically >75 mmHg) where there is rarely enough additional volume to cause an increase in pulmonary pressures or left heart dilatation (Fig. 17-8).
- "Non-restrictive" VSDs are characterized by large defects with low peak velocity/gradient noted on spectral Doppler (typically <25 mmHg) suggesting that there is minimal pressure difference between LV and RV.
- This results in a large transmission of volume to the pulmonary circulation and LV, leading to pulmonary vascular remodeling and an increase in resistance and pressure as well as left heart dilatation. Late in the natural history of this disease *Eisenmenger's syndrome* may occur.

---

- **Key Point:** *Significant VSD shunt leads to LV, not RV, volume overload.*

### Surgical repair
- Patch repair of VSD

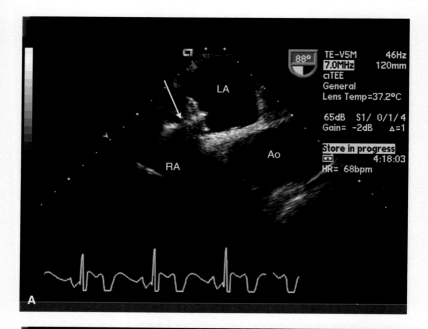

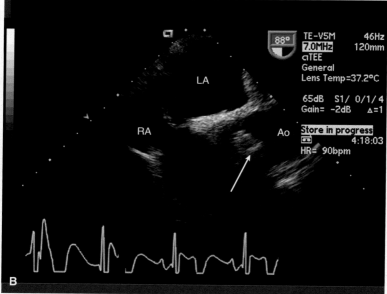

Figure 17-5. TEE 90-degree view of interatrial septum during placement of the clam-shell occluder device. **A:** Shows the occluder positioned across the interatrial septal defect and still attached to the guiding catheter (*arrow*). **B:** A few minutes later after occluder release the device has migrated through the LA and LV to the aorta (*arrow*).

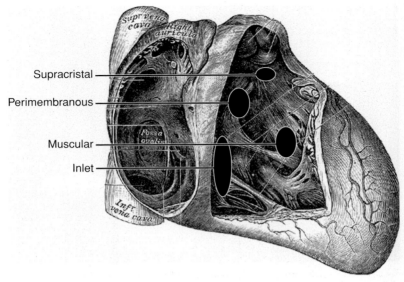

**Figure 17-6.** Anatomic distribution of VSD as seen from the right ventricle. (Adapted from Gray, H. *Anatomy of the Human Body*, 20th ed. Philadelphia: Lea & Febiger, 1918.)

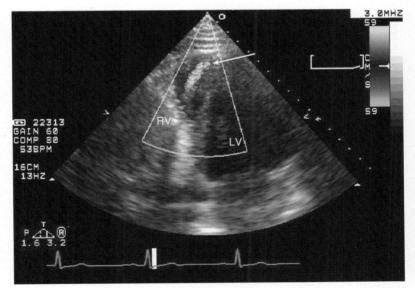

**Figure 17-7.** Off-axis A4C tilted toward the apex to reveal a congenital apical VSD with L→R flow (*arrow*) on color Doppler in a 23-year-old male with a loud systolic murmur.

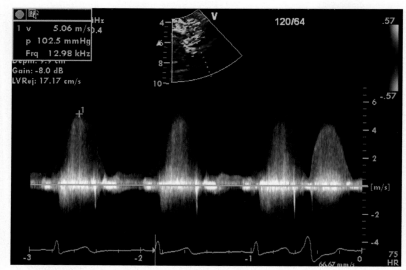

**Figure 17-8.** Systolic flow velocity seen on continuous-wave Doppler with a peak velocity (~5 m/s) and gradient (~103 mmHg) suggestive of a restrictive VSD.

### Echocardiography

- The PSAX at the aortic valve level is a key view to differentiate between perimembranous and supracristal VSD (Fig. 17-9).
- Muscular VSDs are best seen in the A4C and subcostal views. Because of the complex path of these VSDs "off-axis" imaging is often required. They may be **easily missed**.
- Usually associated with other anomalies (patent ductus arteriosis [PDA], ASD, coarctation, tetralogy of Fallot, truncus, and transposition of the great arteries). 25% to 30% occur as isolated defects.
- Evaluate LV dilatation, size of defect in systole and gradient across defect as well as presence of pulmonary hypertension.
- Perimembranous VSD may be partially covered by the septal TV leaflet while supracristal VSD may be partially covered by an aortic leaflet leading to valvular regurgitation.
- Gerbode effect describes flow from the LV to RA through a perimembranous defect and an apical positioned septal leaflet of the TV.
- Postoperatively evaluate the VSD patch for residual shunt.

### C. PDA

- Persistent patency of the ductus arteriosus (present in fetal circulation) connecting the aorta and main PA.
- Arises from the anterior surface of the proximal descending thoracic aorta, distal to the origin of left subclavian artery and enters the main PA.
- The ductus usually functionally closes within 12 to 72 hours of delivery and undergoes complete closure within 3 weeks in term newborn infants.

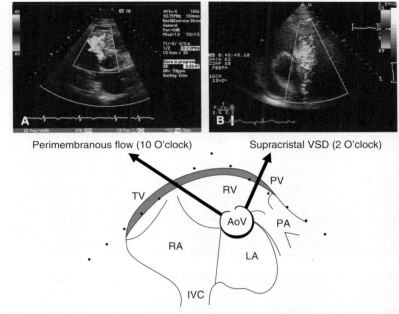

**Figure 17-9.** The central cartoon demonstrates how the direction of the VSD jet in the PSAX view at the aortic level differentiates between **(A)** perimembranous VSD and **(B)** supracristal VSD.

- Most large PDAs are repaired in childhood and usually unrepaired PDAs seen in adulthood are small and insignificant. Large, unrepaired defects eventually lead to Eisenmeinger's syndrome.

### Hemodynamics
- Shunt direction and volume depend on the relative resistance to flow in each pathway normally resulting in **L→R shunting** and LV volume overload and pulmonary hypertension if significant (like VSD).
- **Continuous shunt flow** is seen because of the large pressure difference between the aorta and PA and is noted on auscultation as a continuous machinery grade murmur.
- PASP can be estimated if the SBP is known ($PASP = SBP - 4V_{PDA}^2$).

### Surgical repair
- Closure is most commonly performed as a catheter intervention with surgery reserved for large or complex ductal anatomy.

### Echocardiography
- Evaluate size and gradient across the PDA with identification of flow by color Doppler (Fig. 17-10).
- Evaluate for volume and pressure overload by identifying RVH, LA, and LV dilatation and elevated PA pressures.

> - **Key Point:** *Best view to identify and measure velocity of PDA flow is the PSAX view at the level of the aortic valve with probe tilted toward the pulmonic valve and main PA (ductal view).*

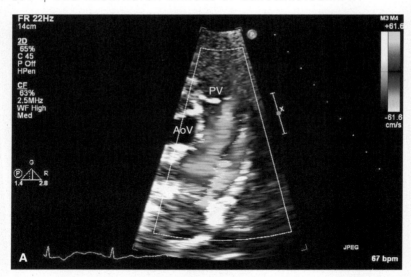

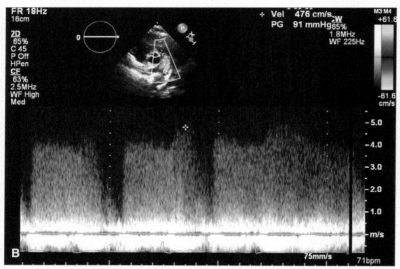

Figure 17-10. **A:** A zoomed PSAX view tilted toward the PV and main PA shows a high velocity jet directed back toward the probe and PV (red jet) consistent with PDA flow. **B:** Continuous-wave Doppler shows classic high velocity continuous flow.

### D. AVCD:

- Failure of embryonic endocardial cushions to meet and form the cardiac crux that normally partitions the center of the heart
- Defects of the cardiac crux
  1. Inlet VSD
  2. Ostium primum ASD
  3. Cleft mitral valve: Commissure between the embryologic anterior and posterior bridging leaflets that cross the septal defect
  4. Abnormal TV

> - **Key Point:** *Considered complete if the above four components are all present and partial, if VSD is absent.*

#### Hemodynamics

- Hemodynamics depend on which components of the defect predominate.
- Combination of ASD and VSD in complete AVCD results in marked volume overload of the pulmonary circulation.
- Abnormalities of AV valves result in significant AV valve regurgitation.

#### Surgical repair

- Patch closure of septal defects and formation of two competent AV valves

#### Echocardiography

See Figure 17-11.

- AV valves are on the same plane!
- Evaluate whether AV connection is single with bridging leaflets and septal attachment or two distinct valves (mitral valve is cleft)
- Evaluate for primum ASD and inlet VSD (A4C)
- LVOT is abnormally elongated ("goose-neck" deformity) and obstruction may be present
- Evaluate PA pressures and evidence for RVH
- Look for other anomalies (PDA, coarctation, hypoplasia of right and left ventricles)
- Post surgery evaluate patch repair for residual shunts and valve repair for regurgitation

## II. OBSTRUCTIONS

### A. Bicuspid aortic valve

- Most common cause of congenital AS (95% of cases). Unicuspid valve is rare.
- Involves fusion of non and right coronary cusps resulting in right and left leaflets or right and left coronary cusps resulting in anterior and posterior leaflets (Fig. 17-12).
- A raphe or line of fusion between the two cusps is often seen and gives the valve a "tricuspid appearance" when viewed in diastole.

> - **Key Point:** *Evaluation of number of cusps should be performed in the PSAX in systole where a bicuspid valve gives an ellipsoid rather than triangular opening.*

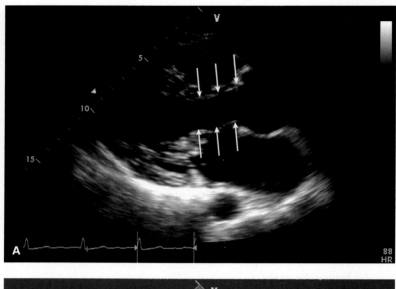

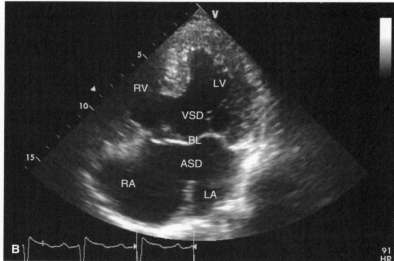

**Figure 17-11.** Characteristic findings suggestive of AVCD. **A:** "Goose-neck" deformity or abnormal elongation of the LVOT seen in the PLAX (*arrows*). **B:** Complete AVCD seen in the (A4C) with large primum ASD and inlet VSD with common bridging AV leaflets (BL).

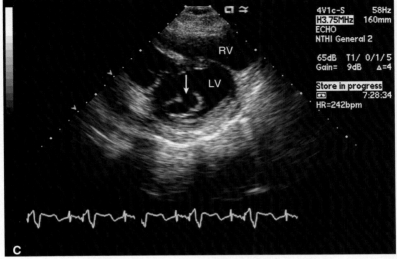

**Figure 17-11.** (*Continued*) **C:** PSAX showing "cleft" mitral valve (*arrow*) in patient with partial AVCD.

- Calcification and fibrosis occur leading to stenosis (more common in anterior–posterior leaflet orientation).
- Because of disproportionate leaflets there is restriction of the opening orifice and eccentric AR secondary to malcoaptation.
- Aortic root dilatation occurs secondary to weakening of the aortic wall.

**Surgical repair**
- Valve replacement when stenosis or regurgitation is severe.

**Echocardiography**
- Bicuspid valve domes in systole because of leaflet restriction and may have prolapse and eccentric regurgitation in diastole because of disproportionate leaflets (PLAX).
- Ellipsoid opening in systole (PSAX).
- Evaluate gradients from multiple views especially because of eccentric opening and aortic jet.
- Measure aortic root diameter and evaluate proximal descending thoracic aorta for coarctation.

B. **Cor triatriatum and congenital mitral stenosis**
- Cor triatriatum and congenital MS are very rare congenital disorders that have usually been surgically corrected by adulthood, unless mild in severity (Fig. 17-13).
- Cor triatriatum describes the division of the LA into two chambers (distal chamber where pulmonary veins enter LA and proximal LA and LA appendage.
- Congenital MS describes a broad range of disorders causing obstruction at the valvular level that include parachute MV and double-orifice MV (Fig. 17-14).

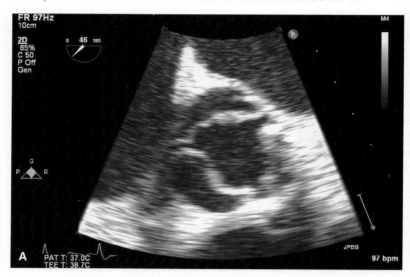

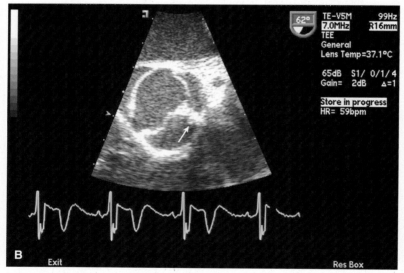

Figure 17-12. TEE short axis of the aortic valve showing: (A) normal triangular opening of a tri-leaflet valve; (B) ellipsoid opening of a bicuspid valve with fusion of the right and left cusps (raphe seen, *arrow*).

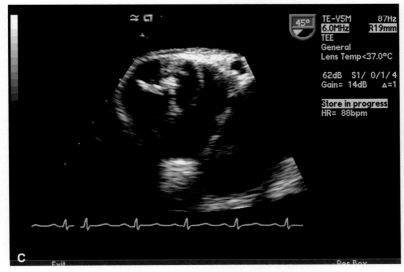

**Figure 17-12.** (*Continued*) **(C)** Unicuspid aortic valve with slit-like opening.

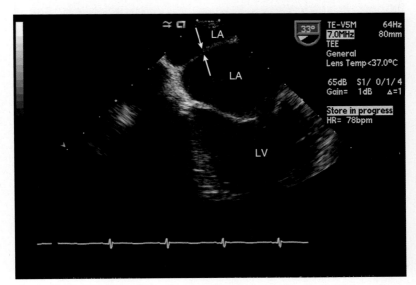

**Figure 17-13.** TEE "Home" view showing cor triatriatum membrane in the LA (*arrows*) separating the pulmonary veins from the proximal LA (MV and LA appendage).

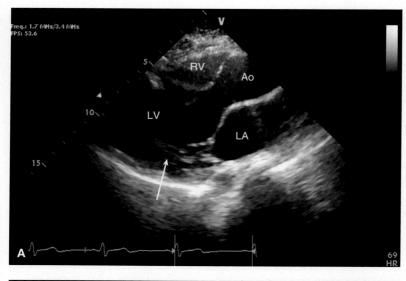

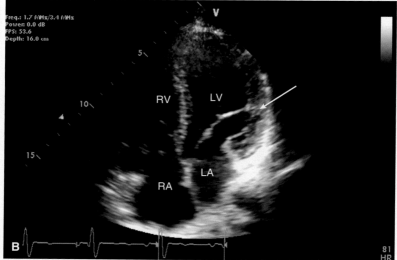

**Figure 17-14.** (A) PLAX and (B) A4C view showing tethering of the mitral leaflet to a single papillary muscle (*arrow*) restricting the opening orifice as can be seen in (C) the PSAX consistent with parachute MV.

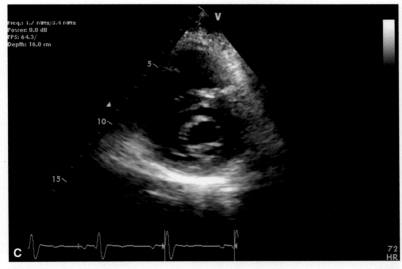

**Figure 17-14.** (*Continued*)

## C. Aortic coarctation

- Congenital obstructive lesion that accounts for 5% to 8% of CHD
- Occurs distal to the origin of the left subclavian artery at the site of the aortic ductal attachment (ligamentum arteriosum)
- **50% of patients with coarctation have bicuspid aortic valve**

### Hemodynamics

- Obstruction of the aorta leads to increased afterload for LV and maldistribution of flow with the proximal/upper segment of the aorta receiving blood flow from LV and lower portions of the body distal to the obstruction having diminished flow/pressure.
- **Collateral flow develops via mammary and intercostal arteries** and may mask the severity of obstruction between upper and lower segments.
- Results in **arterial hypertension.**

### Surgical repair

- Involves resection of narrowed aortic segment and reanastamosis
- May be treated by angioplasty with or without stenting especially in the setting of recoarctation or residual stenosis

### Echocardiography

- Doppler examination is essential and should be directed at the descending aorta in the area of coarctation resulting in a **classic sawtooth flow pattern (elevated peak systolic velocity and diastolic run-off if significant collateral circulation present)** (Fig. 17-15)

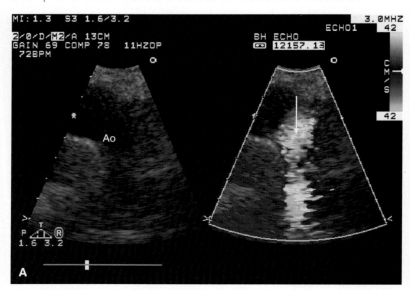

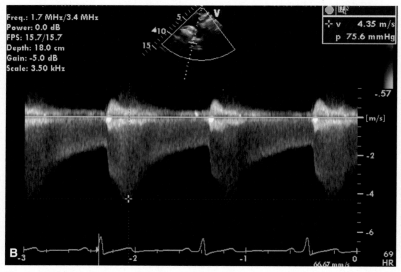

Figure 17-15. **A:** Suprasternal notch view with turbulence and flow acceleration (*arrow*) secondary to narrowing of the proximal descending aorta. **B:** Classic "shark-tooth" spectral Doppler demonstrating increased peak velocity and slow diastolic decrease in velocity consistent with aortic coarctation where significant collateral circulation is present.

- Dual velocity envelopes can be seen representing pre and post coarctation blood flow velocities.
- Evaluate for associated anomalies (bicuspid aortic valve, PDA).
- Postoperative evaluation may show residual stenosis or recoarctation as evidenced by increased peak velocities and turbulence in the proximal descending thoracic aorta. Diastolic run-off may or may not be seen dependent on the presence of collateral flow.

---

- **Key Point:** *Shone's complex describes the presence of multiple left-sided obstructive lesions (congenital MS, subaortic, aortic or supravalvular stenosis, aortic coarctation).*

---

## III. TRANSPOSITION OF THE GREAT ARTERIES

### A. D-TGA

- **Abnormal ventricular–arterial connection**, atrio-ventricular concordance with ventriculo-arterial discordance of aorta to RV and PA to LV

**Hemodynamics/physiology**

**Prerepair**

- A **parallel circulation** is formed with two closed circuits: The systemic circuit venous blood returns from the IVC/SVC to the RV and then recirculates through the aorta and systemic circulation back to the IVC/SVC; the pulmonic circuit oxygenated blood returns from the pulmonary veins to the LV and then recirculates in the pulmonary circulation back to the pulmonary veins.
- **Survival prior to surgery is dependent on the presence of a shunt** (ASD, VSD, PDA) that allows mixing of systemic and pulmonary blood.

**Surgical repair**

**Post repair—*atrial switch***

- *Atrial switch* procedures involve creation of a tunnel or **baffle** (Senning operation uses synthetic material, Mustard operation uses bovine pericardial tissue) to redirect blood from the RA→LA and LA→RA connecting the ventricles **in series. The right ventricle remains the systemic ventricle**.

**Post repair—*arterial switch***

```
      ┌─────────────────────────◄──────────────────────────────┐
      │                                                         │
      └──► Pulm veins → LA → LV → AO ──► SVC, IVC → RA → RV → PA ──►
```

- The more recent and preferred Jatene *arterial switch* procedure allows for complete anatomic and physiologic correction. **The left ventricle is now the systemic ventricle.**
- The aorta and pulmonary arteries are excised from their native roots and reimplanted on the opposite roots respectively (i.e., pulmonary native root becomes neo-aortic root and aortic native root becomes neo-pulmonic root).
- The coronary arteries are reimplanted into the neo-aortic root.
- Postoperative complications include ostial coronary artery stenosis, narrowing of the RVOT and supravalvular AS and PS.

**Echocardiography—post repair**
- Normally the PA wraps around the aorta anteriorly with the pulmonic valve in a perpendicular position compared to the aortic valve. With D-TGA the great arteries are parallel (PLAX, PSAX) with the aorta located anteriorly and rightward (D for Dextro) to the centrally located PA (PSAX) (Fig. 17-16).
- ASD, VSD, or PDA patch may be present and residual shunt should be evaluated with color Doppler.
- Patients with *atrial switch procedures* can be identified as having "busy" atria because of the presence of baffles best seen in the PLAX and A4C (Fig. 17-17).
- Evaluate for possible baffle leaks and stenosis using color, pulsed-wave Doppler, and agitated saline injection (A4C).
- **Look for RV dilatation/dysfunction as the RV is the systemic ventricle and will fail over time.**
- Patients with *arterial switch procedures* can be difficult to distinguish from normal patients. Focal "brightness" may be seen at the anastomosis site of the great arteries (just superior to outflow valves). Evaluate for supravalvular stenosis as well as LV regional wall motion abnormalities secondary to coronary artery ostial stenosis.

B. **L-TGA (physiologically corrected transposition)**
  - **Ventricular–arterial discordance and atrio-ventricular discordance ("two wrongs make a right").** The morphologic RV and associated TV located under left atrium on left side of heart and morphologic LV with associated MV located under right atrium on right side of heart.

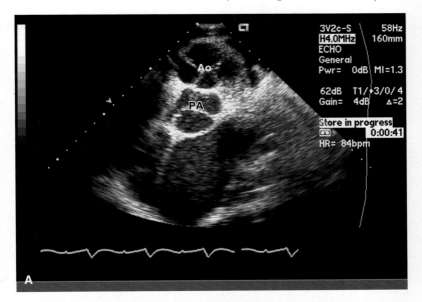

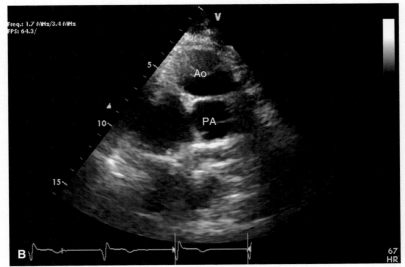

**Figure 17-16.** PSAX demonstrating **(A)** L-TGA with the aorta anterior and toward the left side of the patient compared to the PA and **(B)** D-TGA with the aorta anterior and toward the right side of the patient compared to the PA.

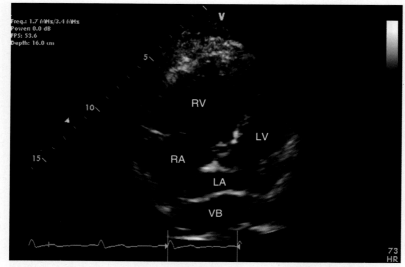

**Figure 17-17.** A4C in patient with D-TGA with history of atrial switch surgery. The venous baffle (VB) can be seen directing blood from the RA to the pulmonic ventricle (morphologic LV).

- Aorta arises from the **morphologic RV (systemic ventricle)** and is parallel (PLAX), anterior, and leftward (L = Levo) of the pulmonary artery (PSAX).

**Hemodynamics**
- Although there is ventricular inversion blood flow through the heart is entirely normal with any derangement of flow secondary to associated defects (VSD, ASD, Ebstein's, aortic stenosis/subaortic stenosis, subpulmonic, pulmonic stenosis [PS], coarctation)

**Echocardiography**
- Identify associated anomalies
- Evaluate outflow valve position and rule out dysplastic AV valves (e.g., Ebstein's anomaly)
- Evaluate RV function and size because as the systemic ventricle it is exposed to systemic pressures and despite marked remodeling will eventually fail

## IV. TETRALOGY OF FALLOT

Tetrad of defining features (Fig. 17-18):
1. RVH
2. VSD
3. Overriding aorta
4. Sub-PS

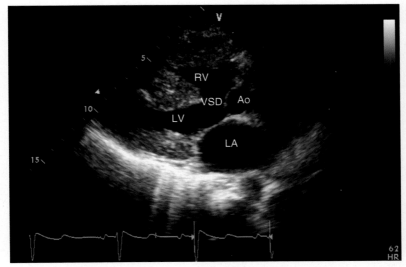

**Figure 17-18.** PLAX of a patient with unrepaired tetralogy of Fallow with large non-restrictive VSD, overriding aorta and marked LVH and RVH.

### Hemodynamics

- **VSD is usually large and non-restrictive** eventually resulting in Eisenmenger's syndrome, RVH and R→L shunting (and cyanosis) if unrepaired. Patients **rarely develop pulmonary hypertension** as subpulmonary and/or pulmonic stenosis (PS) protects pulmonary circuit.
- The greater the percentage of the aorta that overrides the septum the greater the degree of pulmonic obstruction.

### Surgical repair

- Most adults will have had either palliative and/or reparative surgery.
- *Palliative surgeries* are designed to **augment pulmonary blood flow** (which is markedly reduced by PS) and allow normal pulmonary artery development prior to reparative surgery. These include:
  - Blalock–Taussig shunt—subclavian artery to PA anastomosis
  - Waterston shunt—ascending aorta to main or right PA anastomosis
  - Potts shunt—descending aorta to left PA anastomosis
- *Reparative surgery* involves patch closure of the VSD and relieving PS.
- A variety of options to relieve subpulmonic obstruction are available dependent on the clinical presentation and anatomy and may involve resection of subpulmonic muscle bundles, subpulmonic or transannular patch, PV valvotomy or replacement (homograft or bioprosthetic) or Rastelli procedure (conduit from RV to PA).
- Transannular patch repair results in severe PR, RV volume overload, and failure. A limited patch repair with the "trade-off" of residual stenosis may also be performed.

**Echocardiography**
- In the postoperative patient evaluate for residual VSD shunt and subpulmonic obstruction
- After transannular patch or pulmonic valvotomy evaluate degree of PR and RV size and function
- Evaluate conduit flow and peak velocities after Rastelli procedure

## V. TRUNCUS ARTERIOSUS

- Origin of single great artery from the heart which then gives rise to both PA and aorta
- Absence of pulmonary valve
- Cardiac anatomy similar to tetralogy of Fallot with a large perimembranous VSD and overriding great vessel
- The "truncal" valve is often dysplastic with varying degrees of cusp stenosis and insufficiency

**Surgical repair**
- This involves separation of PAs from aorta and placement of an extra **cardiac conduit from RV to PA with VSD closure**. RV to PA conduit will require multiple reoperations as the patient grows.

**Hemodynamics**
- Truncal valve stenosis may result in hypertrophy of both ventricles while truncal valve insufficiency leads to dilatation

**Echocardiography**
- Differentiating truncus from tetralogy may be difficult in undiagnosed cases
- Evaluate anatomy and branching of great artery
- Evaluate truncal valve(s) with careful examination of number of leaflets, degree of stenosis, and insufficiency.

## VI. EBSTEIN'S ANOMALY

- Abnormality of the TV in which the septal and posterior leaflets are markedly apically displaced and the anterior leaflet is elongated ("sail-like") and attached to the RV free wall.
- TV coaptation is apically displaced causing significant regurgitation and "atrialization" of the RV.
- Typically associated with interatrial communication (ASD, PFO).
- Surgical repair when appropriate includes reconstruction or replacement of the TV. The Fontan procedure is primarily done in children who have significant symptoms secondary to hypoplasia of the RV from marked TV displacement, creating single ventricle physiology (see below).

**Hemodynamics**
- The severity of clinical presentation depends on what proportion of the RV remains functional (not "atrialized") and if significant TR causing RV volume overload is present.

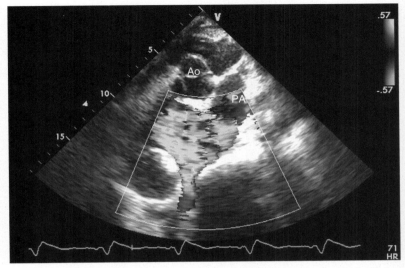

**Figure 17-19.** Off-axis PSAX view with color Doppler demonstrating flow in the Fontan conduit, behind the LA, directing caval blood to the PA.

- Most patients have at least moderate TR secondary to malcoaptation.
- A small RV has diminished filling and contractile capacity leading to right heart failure.
- Associated ASD/PFO allows for R → L shunting leading to hypoxemia when right heart pressures are elevated.

**Echocardiography**

See Chapter 12, Figure 12-1.

- Apical displacement of TV compared to MV >0.8 cm/m$^2$ (indexed to BSA).
- Assess leaflet mobility, attachments of anterior leaflet to RV free wall and size and function of non-affected RV.
- Assess TR severity and pulmonary pressures.
- Identify the presence of interatrial shunts and their significance.

See Figure 17-19, short-axis view of Fontan conduit in a case of hypoplastic right heart.

## VII. FONTAN PROCEDURE FOR SINGLE VENTRICLE PHYSIOLOGY

- This is a palliative procedure for children with single ventricle physiology (e.g., hypoplastic LV or RV, TV atresia) that may occasionally be seen in adults.

- This is performed to reduce the workload of the single ventricle which has to pump blood through the pulmonary and systemic circulation.
- The procedure is performed in two stages with initially blood from the SVC directed to the PAs, which have been disconnected from the pulmonic ventricle (bi-directional Glenn procedure). In the final stage the IVC blood is also directed to the PAs resulting in total caval flow bypassing the pulmonic ventricle (Fontan completion).

# 18 Cardiac Masses

Suzanne V. Arnold

## HIGH-YIELD FINDINGS

- Thrombi usually occur in areas of low flow—for example, alongside an akinetic left ventricular (LV) wall
- Vegetations are typically on the low-pressure side of the valve
- Assess tumors for size, shape, and physiologic significance (i.e., disruption of flow, displacement of normal structures)
- Describe what you see to help develop a differential diagnosis

## COMMON PITFALLS

- Beware of normal variants and pathologic variations of normal structures
- All masses should ideally be seen in more than one plane
- Use color flow and/or intravenous (IV) contrast to ensure mass is not artifactual

## NORMAL VARIANTS AND PATHOLOGIC VARIATIONS OF NORMAL STRUCTURES

### Normal Variants

- **LV false tendons:** Fibromuscular bands that extend across the LV from the septum to the free wall (Fig. 18-1A).
- **Moderator band:** A muscular band that extends across the right ventricle (RV) from the septum to the base of the papillary muscles of the RV.
- Prominent or calcified **papillary muscles** of the mitral valve (MV) or tricuspid valve (TV).
- **Crista terminalis:** A vertical ridge of smooth myocardium that extends between the right side of the orifice of the superior vena cava (SVC) to the right side of the valve of the inferior vena cava (IVC).
- **Eustachian valve:** A valve flap at the distal end of the IVC that directs blood into the right atrium (RA) and toward the interatrial septum. When prominent and filamentous, it is called a Chiari network (Fig. 18-1B).
- **"Coumadin ridge":** Artifact from a prominent fold of tissue that separates the left superior pulmonary vein and the left atrial appendage can be confused on TEE with a thrombus.

### Pathologic Variations of Normal Structures

- Dense mitral annular calcification
- Lipomatous infiltration of the atrial septum (Fig. 18-2)

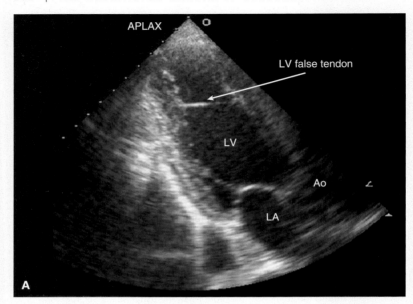

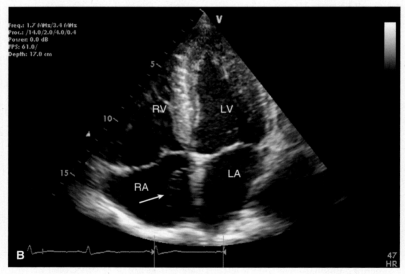

**Figure 18-1. A:** APLAX with bright linear echodensity seen in distal LV consistent with false tendon. **B:** A4C with bright linear echodensity seen in RA consistent with a Chiari network (*arrow*).

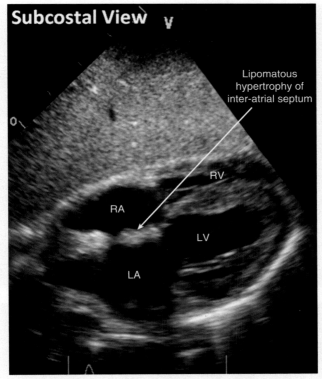

**Figure 18-2.** Subcostal view showing the typical "dumb-bell" appearance of interatrial septal hypertrophy.

- Epicardial fat
- LV trabeculations (e.g., non-compaction, chest wall deformities)
- Lambl's excrescences: Filiform strands (typically small mobile homogeneous echodense structures <1 cm) that originate at valve closure sites. They are usually thought of as a normal variant (found in 70% to 80% of adults), but embolism has been reported (most likely due to superimposed thrombus)

## ARTIFACTS

The use of ultrasound may produce artifacts that give the appearance of masses within the heart. The use of imaging from multiple planes, color Doppler interrogation, and contrast administration will reduce misinterpretation; however, use of alternative imaging modalities may be needed to exclude important pathology. Examples of common ultrasound artifacts are listed below (Fig. 18-3).

*Side-lobe artifact*—secondary, oblique "lobes" of ultrasound energy occur off the main beam axis. In general, because of the lower energy of the side-lobes, this does

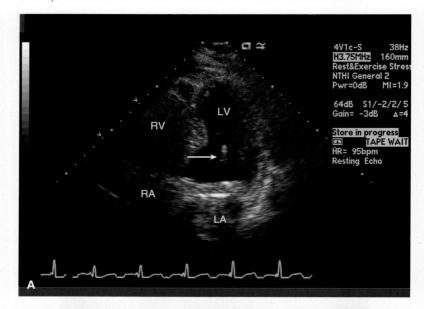

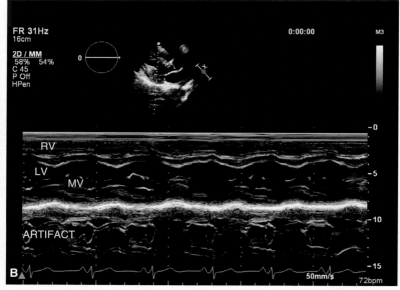

**Figure 18-3.** Ultrasound artifacts: **(A)** Side-lobe artifact places the image of the RV pacing wire in the LV (*arrow*). Note reverberation artifact below mechanical MV, **(B)** PLAX M-mode shows duplication artifact of MV in the echo-free space behind the LV.

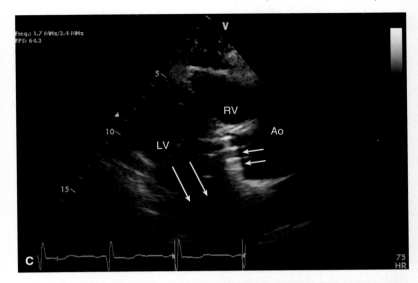

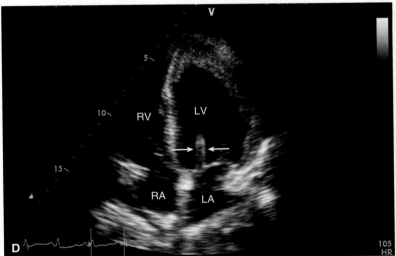

**Figure 18-3.** (*Continued*) (**C**) PLAX in patient with mechanical bi-leaflet valve in the aortic position exhibiting shadowing or attenuation artifact (*long arrows*) as well as reverberation (*short arrows*), (**D**) Comet-tail artifact (*arrows*) in patient with pleural effusions and pulmonary edema (note apical thrombus secondary to hypereosinophilic syndrome).

not commonly affect the image that is displayed. However, occasionally when there is a bright specular reflector (e.g., catheter, wire) detected by the side-lobe, this may be mis-assigned to the main beam and noticeable in the echo-free spaces of the heart or its surroundings.

*Reverberation*—these are secondary reflections that occur when the ultrasound beam meets a bright, fast moving specular reflector that increases the time taken for the signal to return to the transducer. This artifact may be displayed as a trail of bright echoes behind the reflector (e.g., mechanical valve) or as a distinct duplication of the reflector (e.g., MV seen in echo free space posterior to the heart).

*Attenuation*—when the majority of ultrasound energy is reflected back to the transducer because of a strong reflector, there is "shadowing" of the structures behind the reflector and this is displayed as an echo-free space. This may give an appearance of a hypo-echoic mass (e.g., thrombus) and necessitates the use of additional views to find a path that is not "blocked" by the strong reflector to interrogate the area of interest.

*"Comet-tail" artifact*—typically seen in patients with pulmonary edema, pleural effusions and ascites where the ultrasound beam meets an interface between two materials with marked difference in acoustic impedence (i.e., tissue and fluid). This causes a series of micro-reflections on echocardiographic images resembling a "comet-tail."

## TRUE CARDIAC MASSES

### Thrombus

- Intracardiac thrombus comprise one of two varieties: **Thrombus in situ and thrombus in transit.**
- Fresh thrombus is homogenous, has irregular borders, and often has mobile components.
- Old thrombus can be more calcified and is generally less mobile.
- **In situ thrombus occurs at sites of low flow**, thus allowing for clot to form.
  - In the left atrium (LA), this is most often in the LA appendage, best viewed in the apical two-chamber and in the parasternal short-axis view at the level between the mitral and aortic valves. However, this is difficult to visualize adequately with a transthoracic approach and requires transesophageal examination if clinical suspicion is high.
  - In the LV, thrombus is found almost exclusively at the site of a wall motion abnormality. This can be an akinetic, dyskinetic, or aneurysmal segment related to any etiology. Scanning across the apex in multiple, non-foreshortened views and using IV contrast increase sensitivity and specificity for detecting thrombus (Fig. 18-4). An exception to this is Loeffler's endocarditis (i.e., hypereosinophilic syndrome), where LV thrombus occurs without a corresponding wall motion abnormality (Fig. 18-3D).
  - In situ thrombus in the RA and RV is less common often occuring at the site of instrumentation.
  - Thrombus can also occur on foreign bodies in any chamber (e.g., valve prostheses, catheters, pacing wires).
- **Thrombus in transit is typically deep venous thrombus that moves either toward the pulmonary arteries or across an interatrial shunt.** In a patient with a known pulmonary embolus, thrombus in transit can be an indication for thrombolytics or thrombectomy (Fig. 18-5).

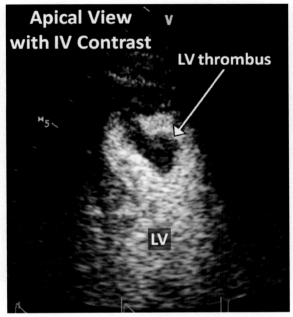

**Figure 18-4.** Zoomed contrast enhanced view of the LV apex showing an echolucent pedunculated mass consistent with thrombus.

## Vegetations

- **Can be infectious or non-infectious. Typically irregularly shaped and attached to the low-pressure side of the valve.**
- Non-infectious vegetations occur due to formation of sterile platelet and fibrin thrombi on cardiac valves in response to trauma, circulating immune complexes, vasculitis, or a hypercoagulable state.
  - Libman–Sacks lesions: Verrucous vegetations associated with systemic lupus erythematosus. These typically have irregular borders, heterogeneous echodensity, and no independent motion and most often involve the basal or mid portions of the MV and aortic valve (AoV). Diffuse valve thickening can be observed and represents the chronic healed phase of the disease process. These are most often clinically silent but valvular abnormalities can occur.
- Infectious vegetations can be bacterial or fungal and are **frequently associated with valvular regurgitation** (see Chapter 14).

## Tumors

- In the case of tumors, it is important to describe the mass and also investigate its physiologic significance.
  - **Pericardial tumors can cause effusion**, impair ventricular filling and lead to cardiac tamponade.

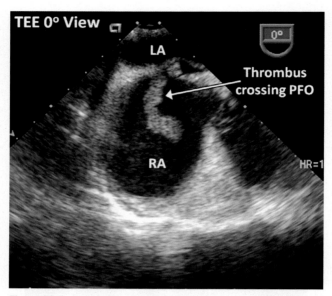

Figure 18-5. An upper-esophageal TEE view of the RA showing a thrombus in transit crossing the interatrial septum.

- **Intracavitary tumors can impair normal flow** through the heart and produce the same physiology as valvular stenosis.
- Extracardiac tumors (such as mediastinal masses) can also displace normal structures and may produce impairment in normal intracardiac flow.

### Benign Tumors

- **Myxomas** account for the majority of benign cardiac tumors. These are most often single masses that arise from the fossa ovalis of the interatrial septum and protrude into the **LA (75% of cases)** (Fig. 18-6).
  - Often are heterogeneous and have an irregular shape.
  - Myxomas are often asymptomatic—found incidentally on imaging—but can produce constitutional symptoms or symptoms from significant impairment to ventricular filling (i.e., "pseudo MS").
- **Papillary fibroelastomas** are the most common primary tumors of the cardiac valves. They most typically are found on the MV and AoV, although they can also be subvalvular or rarely attached to the ventricular free wall. They are usually <1 cm in diameter, pedunculated with high-frequency oscillations during the cardiac cycle, and may appear "frond-like."
- Other benign cardiac tumors include lipomas, rhabdomyomas, and hemangiomas.

### Malignant Tumors

- **Nonprimary cardiac tumors are far more common than primary cardiac tumors.**
- Tumors can involve the heart through direct extension, hematogenous spread, lymphatic spread, or intracavitary extension from the IVC.
- Cardiac involvement from metastatic malignancies most often involves the pericardium and epicardium, presenting as pericardial effusion.

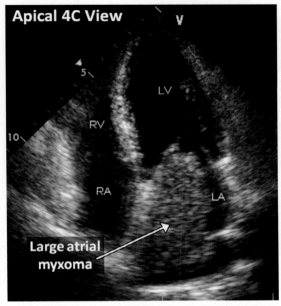

**Figure 18-6.** Apical 4C view showing a large obstructing left atrial myxoma extending from the interatrial septum and filling the mitral valve inflow area.

- **Lung, breast, and hematologic malignancies** comprise the majority of cardiac metastases.
- **Melanoma** has the highest rate of pericardial metastases (Fig. 18-7).
- **Renal cell carcinoma** (and less commonly uterine leiomyoma or hepatoma) **can extend from the kidney up through the IVC** and into the RA. This can appear similar to a thrombus in transit (Fig. 18-8).
- Primary malignant tumors are exceptionally rare, but when they occur, they are most often sarcomas. These are usually intramural, involve any cardiac chamber, grow rapidly, and are destructive (can even cause myocardial rupture). They are associated with a high mortality.

## Establishing a Differential Diagnosis

When an intracardiac mass is seen, describing what you see is the most important step to developing a differential diagnosis—establishing a definitive diagnosis may not always be possible. Describe the following:

- **Location:** Where is the mass attached: pericardial, intramural, intracavitary, valvular
- **Mobility:** Mobile versus sessile, independent or dependent movement with cardiac cycle
- **Visual appearance:** Solid versus hollow, homogeneous versus heterogeneous, echogenic (bright) versus echolucent (dark), irregular versus regular borders, linear versus globular
- **Effect on other structures:** Impairment in chamber filling, valvular stenosis or regurgitation

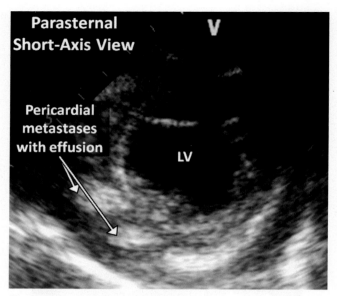

**Figure 18-7.** Parasternal short-axis view of the LV showing bright ovoid echodensities in the pericardial space found to be metastatic breast cancer.

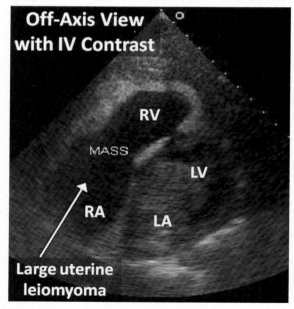

**Figure 18-8.** Off-axis apical four-chamber view that is contrast enhanced showing a large filling defect extending from the RA to the RV that was found to be a uterine leiomyoma.

# 19 Cardiac Manifestations of Systemic Illness

Mohammed K. Saghir, Thomas K. Kurian, and Daniel H. Cooper

## AMYLOIDOSIS

### Classifications

- **Primary**—most common, results from plasma cell dyscrasia and accumulated light chain protein. Cardiac involvement is common with mean survival of 4 months following development of heart failure.
- **Secondary**—amyloid fibrils result from accumulation of acute phase reactant, serum amyloid A. This is often secondary to underlying chronic inflammatory conditions.
- **Hereditary**—secondary to mutations in apolipoprotein I and transthyretin (TTR). Autosomal dominant. Can result in heart failure.
- **Senile**—age related, secondary to accumulation of wild-type transthyretin. Can have significant cardiac involvement. Generally less aggressive than AL.
- **Atrial**—related to age and valvulopathy. Protein is atrial natriuretic peptide and released in response to wall stretch. Uncertain clinical significance.
- **Hemodialysis**—related to accumulation of B2-microglobulin in long-term hemodialysis patients.

### Echocardiographic Findings

See Figure 19-1.

- Early manifestations include progressive diastolic dysfunction and increasing biventricular wall thickness. The LV cavity is normal to slightly reduced in size though it may become dilated late in the disease.
- A granular **"sparkling"** pattern may be noted in the myocardium. Given new harmonic imaging this is not specific for cardiac amyloidosis and can be seen in severe hypertensive heart disease, hypertrophic cardiomyopathy, and glycogen storage disease.
- Amyloid deposits on cardiac valves with **valvular thickening and insufficiency**.
- Advanced cardiac involvement from amyloid may show LV dilatation, LV failure, biventricular thickening, **atrial septal thickening** (specific for amyloid), biatrial dilation, and pericardial effusion.
- Restrictive mitral filling pattern with markedly reduced mitral annular peak velocities.

- **Key Point:** *Atrial septal infiltration/thickening is specific for cardiac amyloidosis in the correct clinical picture and in combination with other suggestive echocardiographic findings.*

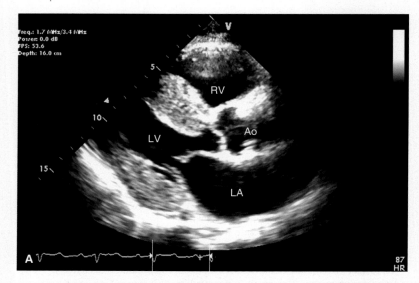

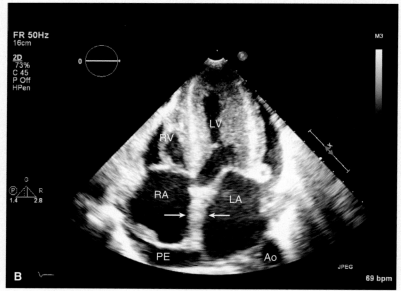

**Figure 19-1.** Patient with amyloid heart disease. **(A)** PLAX and **(B)** A4C shows biatrial enlargement marked LVH with "granular" appearance as well as interatrial septal infiltration (*arrows*).

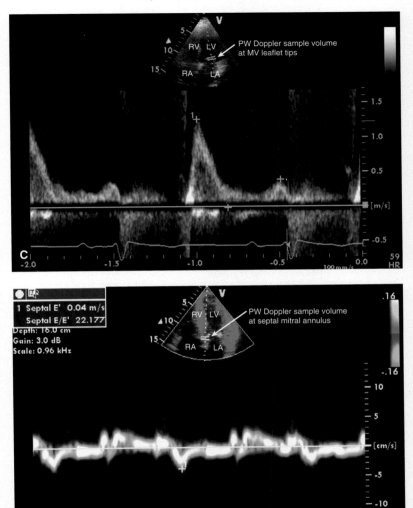

Figure 19-1. (*Continued*) (**C**) Restrictive mitral inflow pattern as well as (**D**) marked reduction in peak tissue Doppler velocity of the mitral annulus.

## CARCINOID

### Background

- Slow growing neuroendocrine tumor often arising from enterochromaffin cells in the gastrointestinal tract. Cardiac involvement occurs following metastasis to the liver and exposure of the heart to active substances such as serotonin and bradykinin. Generally symptoms are **limited to the right heart** as the lungs clear carcinoid-related substances.

### Echocardiographic Findings

See Figure 19-2.

- Carcinoid substances cause valvular thickening and restricted leaflet movement resulting in a **"club"-like appearance of the TV leaflets** with severe TR and variable stenosis. The pulmonic valve may be similarly affected. These valvular changes lead to RV volume overload and eventually failure.
- Subcostal views may reveal liver metastases. Check for hepatic vein systolic flow reversal in this view as a marker of severe TR.
- Rarely, myocardial metastases may be seen.

> - **Key Point:** *Left-sided valvulopathy may occur in a patient with carcinoid disease if an intracardiac right-to-left shunt is present.*

## HYPEREOSINOPHILIC SYNDROME

### Background

- Proliferative disorder characterized by a peripheral eosinophilia (>1500 eosinophils/mm$^3$) of at least 6 months and organ involvement, without any identifiable etiology. Organ dysfunction arises from eosinophilic infiltration and consequent fibrosis. Although several systems can be affected, **mortality is often secondary to myocardial fibrosis and heart failure**.

### Echocardiographic Findings

See Figure 19-3.

- Echocardiographic findings may involve one or both ventricles. Endomyocardial fibrosis shows a predilection for the **LV apex and inflow areas**. Apical obliteration with **LV thrombus** can be seen. The thrombus is in general hypoechoic with punctate calcification.

> - **Key Point:** *Patients with hypereosinophilic syndrome may develop apical thrombus despite normal underlying myocardial contractility. This is an exception to the rule that thrombus forms adjacent to an akinetic or aneurysmal myocardial segment.*

- Basal ventricular hypercontractility may be seen (Merlon's sign).
- Papillary muscle involvement can cause significant mitral valve regurgitation. Inferolateral wall thickening can be noted and autopsy series suggest the possibility of adhesion of the MV leaflet to the inferolateral wall—contributing to MR.
- Tricuspid involvement with concomitant regurgitation may also occur.
- Advanced cases may demonstrate nearly obliterated ventricles with restrictive filling and marked biatrial enlargement.

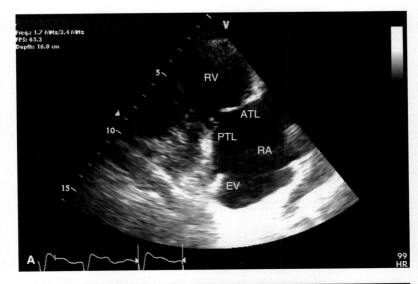

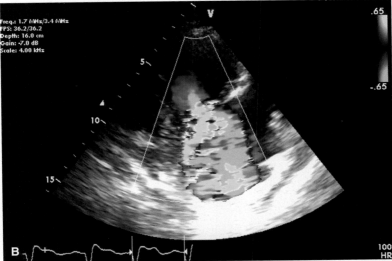

Figure 19-2. Patient with carcinoid heart disease. (A) Parasternal RV inflow view shows shortened, thickened, "club-like" posterior (PTL) and anterior (ATL) TV leaflets with (B) severe TR seen on color Doppler. (ev, eustachian valve) (*continued*)

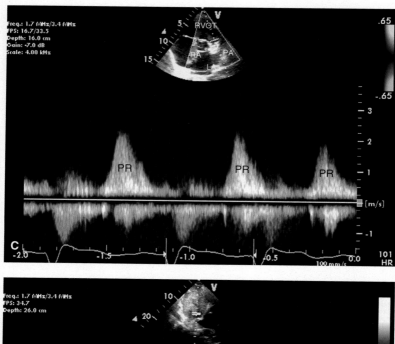

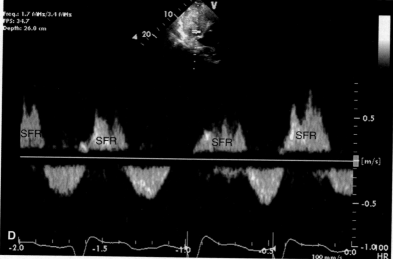

**Figure 19-2.** (*Continued*) (**C**) CW Doppler across the pulmonic valve in the PSAX view shows a dense, diastolic jet with a short deceleration time consistent with severe PR. (**D**) Hepatic Doppler exhibits systolic flow reversal suggestive of severe TR.

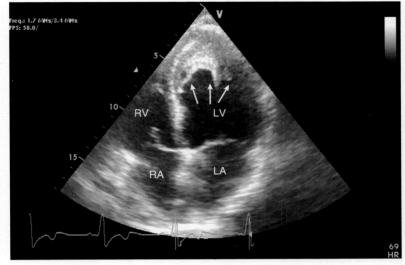

Figure 19-3. A4C in patient with hyperesosinophilic syndrome shows obliteration of the LV apex by thrombus (*arrows*).

## MARFAN SYNDROME

### Background

- Connective-tissue disorder of the FBN1 gene, which encodes fibrillin-1, a supporting protein for elastin and vascular smooth muscle. Usually autosomal dominant but can be a spontaneous mutation. Involved systems include cardiac, pulmonary (pneumothorax), musculoskeletal, ocular, and neurologic (dural ectasia). Aortic dilatation, dissection, and cardiac valvulopathy are known to also occur.

### Echocardiographic Findings

- Dilatation of the aortic annulus, ascending aorta, and **sinuses of Valsalva** is noted in 60% to 80% of Marfan patients (Fig. 19-4). Aortic dissection may occur secondary to intrinsic wall weakness and dilatation.

## RADIATION INDUCED CARDIOMYOPATHY

### Background

- Mediastinal radiation can damage coronary arteries, valves, pericardium, and myocardium leading to proximal coronary stenosis, pericardial effusion, valvular disease, systolic dysfunction, and restrictive cardiomyopathy. **The time course of cardiac manifestations is variable.**

### Echocardiographic Findings

- Echocardiographic findings in radiation-induced cardiomyopathy are often nonspecific. The systolic and the diastolic dysfunction may occur and can progress to restrictive cardiomyopathy.

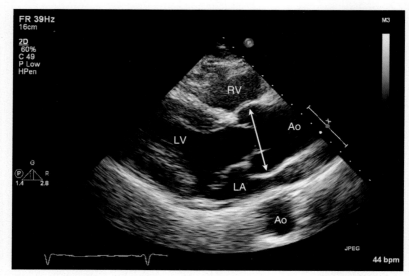

**Figure 19-4.** PLAX in Marfan's patient with dilatation of the sinus of Valsalva (*double-headed arrow*) giving a "pear-shaped" appearance to the aortic root.

• Valvular disease may be seen as **thickening and valvular insufficiency**. The tricuspid valve is particularly affected secondary to its anterior location and proximity to the radiation source.

---

• **Key Point:** *In a patient with generalized thickening and insufficiency of multiple valves, carefully review the clinical history for mediastinal radiation exposure.*

---

## SARCOIDOSIS

### Background

• Systemic inflammatory condition characterized by the formation of non-caseating granulomas. Involvement includes the lungs, heart, skin, and reticuloendothelial system. A higher prevalence of this condition is seen in African Americans. Although cardiac involvement by sarcoid can be asymptomatic, complications include conduction abnormalities, arrhythmias, dilated cardiomyopathy, LV aneurysm, and pericardial effusion.

### Echocardiographic Findings

• Progressive diastolic dysfunction is seen with an initially preserved ejection fraction. Systolic dysfunction occurs late in the disease.

---

• **Key Point:** *Regional areas of myocardial thickening are thought to be secondary to sites of active inflammation and granuloma formation. These eventually progress to fibrosis and focal myocardial thinning especially at the **basal septal and inferolateral walls** (Fig. 19-5). **These look like aneurysmal "bites" out of the myocardium.***

---

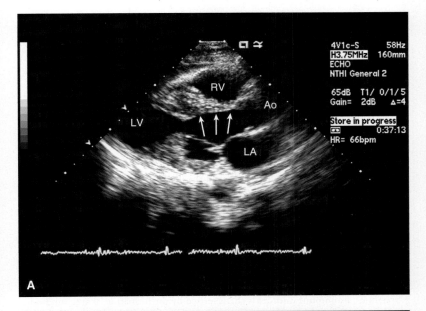

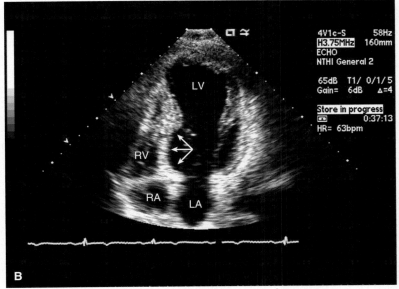

Figure 19-5. Patient with sarcoidosis and (A) basal anteroseptal and (B) inferoseptal aneurysms (*arrows*) secondary to myocardial fibrosis, seen in the PLAX and A4C views respectively.

- Valvular thickening can occur resulting in significant regurgitation.
- Pulmonary hypertension from sarcoidosis may result in RV hypertrophy.

## SCLERODERMA

### Background

- Chronic autoimmune disease is characterized by arteriolar fibrosis and multiorgan involvement. Formerly known as the CREST syndrome (calcinosis, Raynaud's syndrome, esophageal dysfunction, sclerodactyly, and teleangiectasias). Affected organs include the skin, esophagus, lungs, kidneys, and heart.

### Echocardiographic Findings

- Non-specific reduction in the systolic and the diastolic ventricular function is seen with evidence of restrictive cardiomyopathy.
- Pulmonary hypertension and RV dysfunction may result from primary lung disease or secondary LV failure.
- Infrequently, pericardial effusion and pericarditis may be seen.

## SYSTEMIC LUPUS ERYTHEMATOSUS

### Background

- Systemic autoimmune disorder is characterized by the formation of auto-antibodies against certain nuclear antigens. The resultant formation and subendothelial deposition of immune-complexes can cause inflammatory effects in a variety of organ systems, including the heart. Cardiac complications of SLE include valvulitis, vegetations, coronary artery disease, pericarditis, pericardial effusion, and the systolic and the diastolic ventricular dysfunction.

### Echocardiographic Findings

- Valvulitis occurs from a secondary antiphospholipid syndrome. Affected leaflets become thickened and fibrotic resulting in regurgitation.
- **Libman–Sacks vegetations may be noted with valvulitis.** Such vegetations are **irregular** and **cauliflower-shaped** often **<1 cm** in diameter and are heterogenous in appearance. The presence of vegetations may exacerbate regurgitation and can also be **embolic**. The appearance of Libman–Sacks vegetations may be mistaken for infective endocarditis and should be interpreted within the clinical presentation of the patient. **Left-sided valves are affected more frequently than right.**
- **Pericarditis and pericardial effusions** may be seen but rarely have tamponade physiology. Pericardial thickening and constrictive pericarditis is also a rare complication in SLE.

# 20 Transesophageal Echocardiography

Ravi Rasalingam and Anupama Rao

## COMMON INDICATIONS

- Valvular endocarditis
- Cardiac source of embolism
- Mitral/aortic valve disease
- Prosthetic valve disease
- Aortic dissection/aneurysm
- Intracardiac masses

## CONTRAINDICATIONS

- Oro-pharyngeal obstruction
- Esophageal obstruction, that is, spasm, stricture, tumor
- Esophageal injury; that is, laceration, perforation
- High risk of gastroesophageal bleeding; for example, varices, bleeding ulcer
- Prior history of oropharyngeal, esophageal, gastric surgery—discuss with GI/surgeon prior to procedure to define level of risk
- Cervical spine instability
- Severe hypoxemia requiring high-flow oxygen

## KEY VIEWS

- 0 degrees: Mid esophageal view
  - Four-chamber "central" home view
  - Four-chamber "inferior" home view obtained by advancing the probe to show coronary sinus
  - Five-chamber "superior" home view obtained by pulling probe back to show LVOT
- 30 degrees: Mid esophageal view
  - Aortic valve, LAA, LUPV (counterclockwise rotation)
- 60 degrees: Mid esophageal view
  - Bicommissural view: Two-chamber view of LV
  - Clockwise rotation: RV inflow/outflow
- 90 degrees: Mid esophageal view
  - Clockwise rotation: Bicaval view
  - Further clockwise rotation: RUPV
  - Counterclockwise rotation: Two-chamber view of LV, LAA

- 120 degrees: Mid esophageal view
  - Long-axis view of LV
  - Counterclockwise rotation: AoV
- 0 degrees: Transgastric view
  - Short axis of LV at level of MV
  - Short axis of LV at papillary muscle level
- 90 degrees: Transgastric view
  - Two-chamber view of LV
  - Clockwise rotation: RV inflow view
- 120 to 140 degrees: Transgastric view
  - Long axis of LV, AoV
- 0 degrees: Deep-transgastric view
  - Apical portion of LV, flexion to see LVOT, AoV
- Aortic examination at 0 and 90 degrees
  - Descending aorta, arch

## BASIC PRINCIPLES

- **Transesophageal echocardiography (TEE) allows high resolution imaging of posterior cardiac structures and thoracic great vessels closest to the esophagus.**
  - The TEE probe is a long (~100 cm), flexible tube with piezoelectric crystals at its tip capable of high frequency (3 to 7 Hz) imaging.
    - Because of the small depth of imaging using this approach, the highest frequency is most often used to obtain high spatial resolution.
  - The tip of the probe may be bent in an anterograde (flexion) and retrograde (extension) orientation by rotating a large wheel at the base of the probe. The leftward and the rightward movement can also be performed with rotating an adjacent smaller wheel.
    - Levers that lock the wheels and therefore the orientation of the probe are available but in general should not be used in order to minimize potential risk of esophageal trauma.
  - The orientation of the piezoelectric crystal and therefore the imaging plane can be rotated around the long axis of the ultrasound beam by a toggle at the base of the probe. The resulting alteration in angle (in degree increments to a maximum of 180 degrees) is indicated by a semicircle icon on the machine screen.
    - This feature allows multiple planes of a structure to be viewed without moving the probe.
    - At 0 degrees the crystal or imaging plane is horizontal with the patients right side appearing on the left side of the display.
    - As the angle increases the beam rotates in a clockwise fashion. The view at 180 degrees is a mirror image of the 0-degree view.
- **Machine settings:**
  - The probe is inserted into the machine and is selected as the probe for imaging.
  - Typically there is a TEE preset that is customized by the machine vendor. In general, the examiner alters the probe power with higher frequencies used in the esophageal views for high resolution of adjacent cardiac structures. Lower frequencies are used in the transgastric views for improved penetration to see cardiac

structures that are now further from the transducer. Gain settings and focus are altered to optimize the image.

- Acquisition is set to capture number of beats or time, if the triggering EKG is unstable or irregular

## PATIENT EVALUATION AND PREPARATION

- **Adequate patient evaluation and preparation prior to probe intubation reduces procedural complications and inappropriate studies.**
- **In answering the referring physician's question it is important to decide whether TEE, TTE, or a combined approach is most suitable.**
  - TEE affords higher resolution imaging especially of posterior cardiac structures and is superior than TTE for example when evaluating possible valvular endocarditis, left atrial (LA) masses, mitral valve disease, prosthetic valves, or thoracic aortic pathology.
  - There is benefit in a *combined* approach where Doppler-based hemodynamic assessment may be more accurate by a transthoracic echocardiogram (TTE) because of better orientation with blood flow. This data complements the increased anatomic detail provided by TEE.
  - TTE is superior to TEE when imaging structures closer to the chest wall such as the left ventricle (LV) to measure function or assess for apical pathology.
- **Patient preparation includes the following:**
  - In non-emergent cases patients should be NPO for >4 to 6 hours to prevent aspiration. Patients who are intubated should have feeding stopped for this period of time.
  - A history focused on the reason for the study as well as the following elements should be obtained:
    - Recent oropharyngeal, esophageal, or gastric obstruction or bleeding should prompt referral/discussion with gastroenterology prior to TEE
    - A past history of oropharyngeal, esophageal, or gastric surgery that may impact safe passage of the probe
    - Prior history of anesthesia-related complications
    - Medication allergy history
  - Physical examination should assess the following:
    - Current hemodynamic status of the patient
    - Poor dentition, loose teeth, removable bridges
  - **Anesthesia airway score** will help identify patients at high risk of airway complications. This is determined by the amount of space in the posterior pharynx.
  - The following studies and their findings should be reviewed prior to the procedure:
    - Past TTE/TEE studies
    - Other imaging studies pertinent to the indication for TEE
    - Severe anemia (Hb <7 g/dL) in the setting of active bleeding
    - Supratherapeutic INR (>4) should prompt postponement of the procedure or treatment with fresh frozen plasma if urgent to prevent bleeding from contact of the probe with the esophagus
    - Platelet count <40,000, especially if there has been a recent decline should prompt administration of IV platelets to prevent bleeding during the procedure

○ Significant liver dysfunction may affect the pharmacodynamics of sedatives used for the procedure
- **The following procedure-related risks should be explained to the patients in addition to description of the procedure itself prior to consent:**
  - Mortality is close to zero in several large population studies
  - 1 in 10,000 risk of esophageal perforation
  - 3 in 10,000 risk of esophageal bleeding
  - 3 in 1,000 risk of dental injury (higher if poor dentition)
  - 1 in 1,000 risk of severe odynophagia, more commonly mild if present

## TEE Procedure

- A recently placed, functional IV (20 gauge or higher) should be present to allow safe administration of sedation and fluid resuscitation if required.
- Patient vitals (heart rate, blood pressure, oxygen saturation) should be monitored every 3 to 5 minutes during and after the administration of sedation.
- Wall mounted suction via a Yankauer tube should be available to clear the airway of secretions.
- A nurse or anesthesiologist should be present to administer sedation and monitor patient vital signs during and after the procedure. In most cases intravenous opioid and benzodiazepines are used for "conscious sedation." Elderly patients often need only a small dose of these medications, which act in a synergistic manner.

---

- **Key Point:** *To reverse excessive sedation in adults from a benzodiazepine, use Flumazenil IV 0.2 mg and from an opiate use Naloxone IV 0.4 mg. Repeat dosing may be required because of the longer duration of effect of the sedating medication.*

---

- **Key Point:** *A rare, idiosyncratic, paradoxical reaction may occur with benzodiazepines causing the patient to have one of the following responses: (a) uncontrollable weeping, depression; (b) agitation, aggression, disinhibited behavior. This has been mostly described in younger patients and resolves with stopping the administration of the medication.*

---

- **Esophageal Intubation**
  - Dentures/plates are removed from the mouth and the oropharynx is locally anesthetized with topical benzocaine spray and lidocaine gel to reduce the gag reflex. Despite adequate local anesthesia anxious patients may still gag therefore reassurance and a clear explanation of what to expect is important.

---

  - **Key Point:** *Rarely Benzocaine spray can cause methemoglobinemia. This is cyanosis secondary to an increase in the methemoglobin fraction of blood (normal <2%) and subsequent reduction in oxygen carrying capacity. Treatment is IV methylene blue 2 mg/kg.*

---

  - The patient is typically in a left lateral decubitus position with chin tucked to chest (best position to prevent aspiration and align the esophagus for easy intubation). Other positions include the patient sitting up in a 90-degree position with head bent forward. Mechanically ventilated patients are intubated lying flat.
  - A bite-block is placed to protect the probe.

- Ensure that there is no damage to the probe casing and that movement with the wheels at the base and alteration of the transducing beam angle are functional prior to intubation.
- The probe is slightly flexed dependent on the curve of the tongue and the palate. This is advanced to the back and center of the mouth and then straightened and passed into the esophagus.
- NEVER push against resistance.
- If the patient is awake, encourage swallowing when ready to pass the probe into the esophagus.
- Typically the most uncomfortable locations for the patient are when the probe is at the back of the oropharynx, high esophageal position and gastroesophageal junction. Limit time in these areas when possible.

---

- **Key Point:** *Usually assistance with a forward "jaw-thrust" is required to allow easier esophageal intubation of patients with an endotracheal tube, small oropharynx, and/or large tongue. Increased resistance is likely to be felt during intubation; however, care should still be taken not to force movement of the probe into the esophagus. Removal of naso-gastric and oral feeding tubes may aid intubation and image quality. If not removed, the position of these tubes should be checked postprocedure by chest x-ray as movement may occur with manipulation of the TEE probe.*

---

## BASIC VIEWS

- **General Comments**
  - The instructions described are for an operator standing to the patient's left, holding the probe controls with the right hand and the probe near the patient's mouth with the left hand.
  - Most structures can be obtained by movement of the probe itself with use of the wheels at the base of the probe optimizing image definition.
  - Small movements of the probe outside of the patient translate to large movements within the patient at the transducer level.
  - Movements of the probe are made with the hand closest to the patient's mouth.
  - Clockwise rotation of the probe images right heart structures, counterclockwise rotation images left heart structures.
  - Flexion of the probe angles the ultrasound beam superior while extension angles the beam inferior.
  - The operator should rely on the image obtained rather than depth of the probe to produce the views detailed below. If the probe is deeply advanced without producing the expected image consider coiling of the probe (resistance should be felt) or tracheal intubation (associated patient dyspnea, coughing, and hypoxia).
  - Structures of interest should be stored with a focused ultrasound beam at standard and "zoomed" views.
  - For image orientation the left atrium is the most posterior structure and is therefore displayed at the top of the screen closest to the probe.

## BASIC VIEWS

The examination described is a view-based TEE assessment where all structures in a given view are studied. An alternative assessment not described below is a structure-based system where structures of interest are imaged sequentially at different angles.

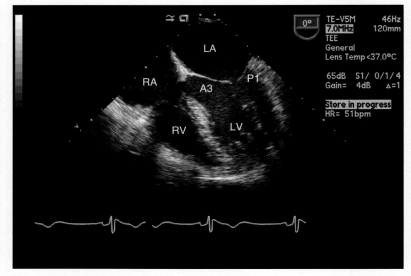

**Figure 20-1.** Home view.

- **Mid esophageal 0-degree view "Home View"**
  - 30 to 40 cm from the incisors with imaging power at 7 MHz and depth set to allow all four cardiac chambers to be seen (Fig. 20-1).
  - Ideally slight extension provides a non-foreshortened view but "contact" with the esophagus may be lost compromising the image. The RV anterior wall and LV inferoseptal and anterolateral walls are seen in this view.
  - Mitral valve anterior leaflet is seen arising from the septum. Mitral valve A3 and P1 cusps seen in *central* "Home View".
  - Advancement of the probe demonstrates the *inferior* "Home View" with A2 and P2 cusps of the mitral valve and the *coronary sinus seen.* Rotation of the probe clockwise at this level shows the septal and anterior tricuspid leaflets.
  - The probe is then pulled back to show the *superior* "Home View" with the *LVOT and aortic valve leaflets visible.* In this higher esophageal position mitral valve A1 and P1 cusps are seen.
- **Mid esophageal 30-degree view**
  - The aortic valve is seen in cross-section at the base of the heart by withdrawing the probe to a higher esophageal position or flexion of the probe tip (Fig. 20-2).
  - The left atrial appendage (LAA) can be evaluated in this higher esophageal position next to the aortic valve. Color Doppler and pulsed-wave Doppler velocities (normal >40 cm/s) should also be obtained.
  - The left superior pulmonary vein is seen by further counterclockwise rotation with color and pulsed-wave Doppler. Pulsed-wave Doppler shows continuous flow (with systolic and diastolic peak velocities) as opposed to Doppler obtained in the LAA.

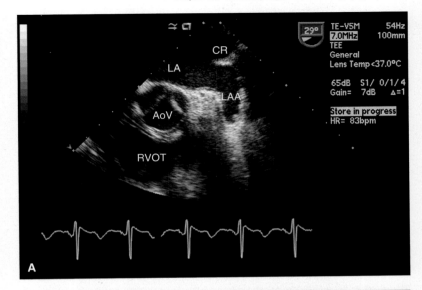

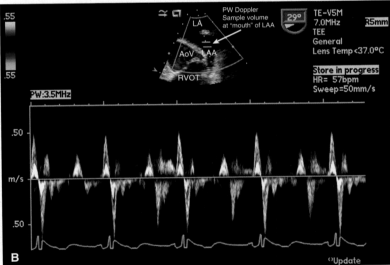

**Figure 20-2.** **A:** Short-axis view of the aortic valve. CR, coumadin ridge; LAA, left atrial appendage; RVOT, right ventricular outflow tract. **B:** Normal pulse-wave Doppler pattern in the left atrial appendage.

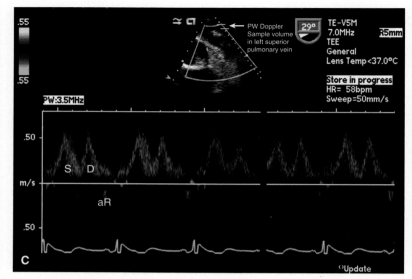

**Figure 20-2.** (*Continued*) **C:** Normal pulse-wave Doppler pattern in the left superior pulmonic vein. S, systolic; D, diastolic; and aR, atrial reversal; pulmonary vein flow.

- **Mid esophageal 60-degree view "Bicommissural View"**
  - Clockwise rotation of the probe shows the RV inflow/outflow view with visualization of the anterior and posterior tricuspid valve leaflets. This view is typically best for obtaining Doppler-based assessment of peak systolic pulmonary pressures from the TR jet (Fig. 20-3).
  - Note, as the piezoelectric crystal moves past 60 degrees a **transition** occurs where the posterior mitral valve leaflet is now displayed on the left and the anterior mitral valve leaflet on the right side of the screen.
  - Counterclockwise rotation develops the bicommissural view so named as the ultrasound beam bisects the "horse-shoe" shaped mitral valve commissures at two locations. This is one reason why multiple regurgitant jets may be noted in this view. From left to right, P1-A2-P3 mitral valve cusps are seen.
  - The mitral subvavular appartus (chordae, papillary muscles) is best assessed in this view.
  - The LAA is reassessed in this view.
- **Mid esophageal 90-degree view "Bicaval View"**
  - The probe is rotated clockwise and withdrawn to demonstrate the interatrial septum (IAS). Color Doppler is used to assess for patent foramen ovale or secundum ASD. Clockwise rotation with deeper probe placement shows the IVC entrance and counterclockwise rotation and withdrawal of the probe shows the SVC. This is especially important in the assessment of sinus venosus ASD and pacing wires and intracardiac catheters (Fig. 20-4).
  - Further clockwise rotation shows the entrance of the right superior pulmonary vein using color Doppler and pulsed-wave Doppler.
  - Counterclockwise rotation and advancement of the probe shows a two chamber view with the anterior and inferior walls of the left ventricle seen. Different depth settings and focus should be used to evaluate the LA, LV, and mitral valve.

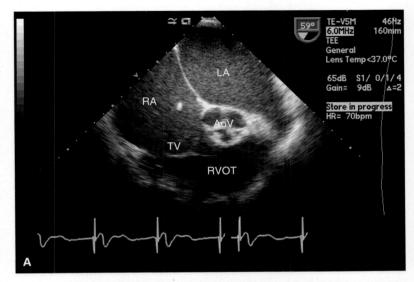

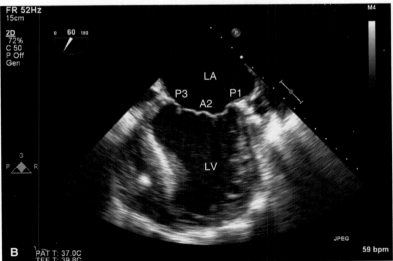

Figure 20-3. **A:** Mid esophageal RV inflow/outflow view. **B:** Mid esophageal mitral bicommissural view.

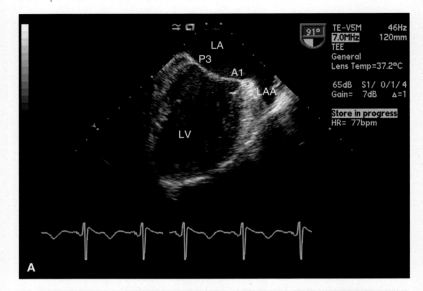

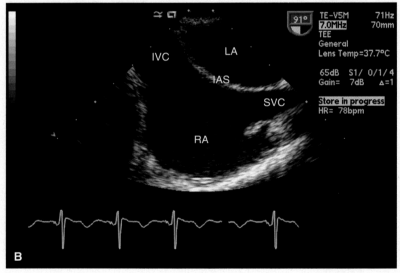

Figure 20-4. A: 90-degree two-chamber view (LA and LV). B: 90-degree bicaval view.

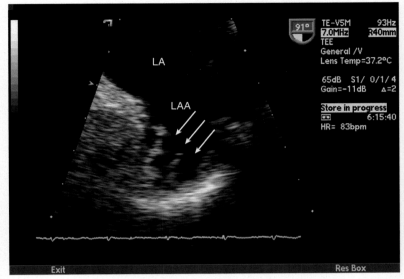

**Figure 20-5.** Pectinate muscles (normal finding, arrows) projecting from the apex of the LAA.

- Mitral valve P3-A1 cusps seen
- The LAA is reassessed in this view

---

- **Key Point:** *The LAA should be assessed in multiple non-foreshortened views as often times it is multi-lobed. Do not mistake the fine finger-like projections at the apex for thrombi. These are pectinate muscles and represent normal LAA anatomy (Fig. 20-5). Also, fibrinous material lying in the transverse sinus behind the LAA may also be occasionally mistaken for LAA thrombus.*

---

- **Mid esophageal 120-degree view "Long-Axis View"**
  - Inferolateral and anteroseptal walls of LV seen
  - P2–A2 mitral valve cusps seen
  - The aortic valve is seen with counterclockwise rotation (typically non and right coronary cusps) (Fig. 20-6)
  - The aortic root (sinus of Valsalva, sinotubular junction, and proximal ascending aorta) is assessed by withdrawing the probe to a higher esophageal position. The angle should be reduced to ~100 degrees with rotation and slight flexion to visualize the ascending aorta
- **Transgastric 0-degree view**
  - The probe is advanced without resistance into the stomach. The ultrasound power is decreased to 5 MHz to allow better penetration and the imaging depth is increased for better visualization.
  - Advancing and flexing the probe just past the gastroesophageal junction the mitral valve *en face* view is seen with all cusps visualized (note the posterior leaflet is closest to the probe). This is a good view for confirmation of the location of a regurgitant jet. Clockwise rotation at this level shows the coronary sinus (Fig. 20-7).

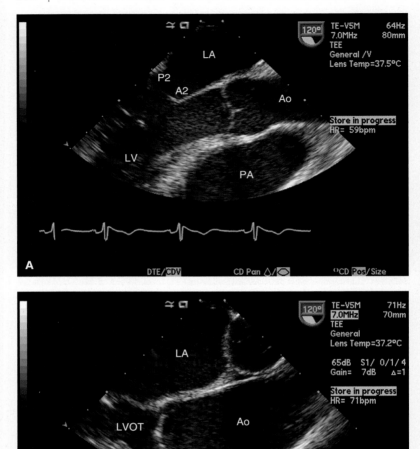

**Figure 20-6. A:** 120-degree LV long-axis view. **B:** Evaluation of aortic root by withdrawing the probe in the LV long-axis view.

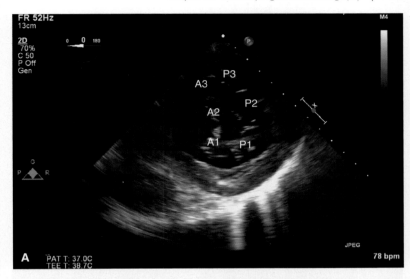

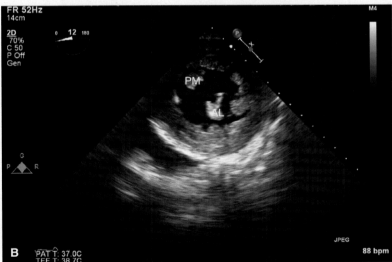

**Figure 20-7. A:** Transgastric LV short-axis view at the level of the mitral valve. **B:** Transgastric LV short-axis view at the papillary muscle level. (PM, posteromedial; AL, anterolateral papillary muscles.)

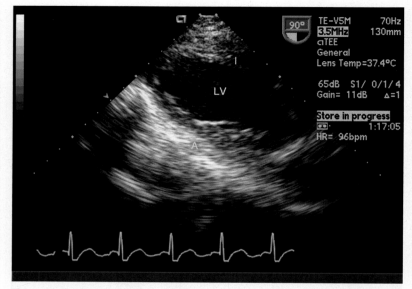

**Figure 20-8.** Transgastric 90-degree view of the LV (anterior and inferior walls).

- Deeper probe placement shows the cross-section of the LV at the mid-papillary muscle level. Flexion again brings the mitral valve into view and subvalvular apparatus while extension or advancing the probe shows the apex of the LV. This is a good view to assess LV wall motion and interventricular septal motion or defects
- Clockwise rotation shows the *en face view of* the tricuspid valve
- **Transgastric 90-degree view**
  - Left ventricular anterior and inferior walls and mitral valve are seen (Fig. 20-8).
  - Clockwise rotation shows the tricuspid valve in the RV inflow view with posterior and anterior leaflets seen.
  - **Transgastric 140-degree view**
  - A long-axis view of the left ventricle is seen particularly for assessment of the aortic valve.
- **Deep transgastric 0-degree view**
  - The probe is advanced until the apical portion of the LV is seen. The large wheel at the base is then rotated to provide maximal flexion. The probe is carefully withdrawn until the left ventricular outflow tract and aortic valves are seen.
  - This is the best view for Doppler alignment for aortic valve stenotic and regurgitant jets.
- **Aortic examination at 0 and 90 degrees**
  - The probe is rotated posteriorly and the imaging depth is reduced and power increased to 7 MHz for high-resolution visualization of the thoracic aorta. If the probe is deep often times withdrawal of the probe is required to see the thoracic aorta.
  - As the probe is withdrawn 0-degree and 90-degree images are taken to evaluate aortic size and presence of pathology. If pathology such as aortic atheroma or hematoma is noted views at both orientations with and without color Doppler are encouraged to best define the structures seen.

- A high esophageal view of the aorta and PA can be seen prior to the aortic arch views (Fig. 20-9).
- At the aortic arch the arch vessels and the right pulmonary artery are seen.
- Color Doppler and pulsed-wave Doppler are used to assess aortic flow.

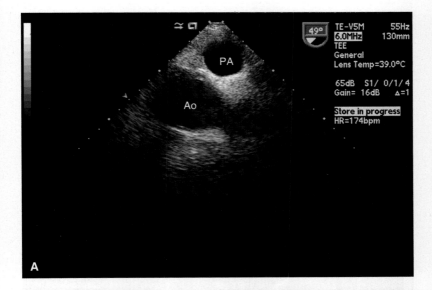

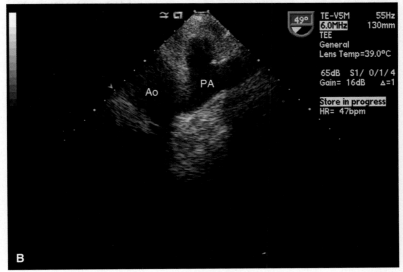

Figure 20-9. (A) High esophageal views of the thoracic aorta and PA, with clockwise rotation of the probe showing the main PA bifurcation (B).

## ADDITIONAL COMMENTS ON DOPPLER EVALUATION

• **Key Point:** *Pulsed-wave Doppler in the proximal descending thoracic aorta should be performed in patients with moderate or greater aortic valve regurgitation to assess for holodiastolic flow reversal.*

• **Key Point:** *For PISA assessment of mitral regurgitation severity the Nyquist baseline is moved down (opposite to TTE) to increase or optimize visualization of the mitral regurgitant flow convergence distance. Remember always move the baseline in the direction of flow of interest to allow for earlier aliasing and increased PISA radius for measurement.*

• **Key Point:** *Reducing imaging depth and color box sector width will help acquire images at correct Nyquist limits and detect higher velocity jets with pulsed-wave Doppler.*

## MINI ATLAS OF TEE IMAGES

### Mitral Valve

See Figures 20-10 and 20-11.

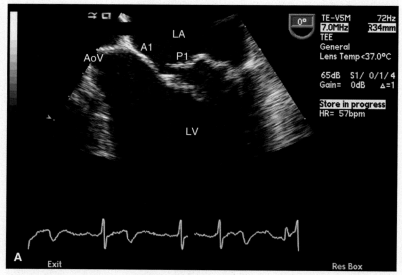

**Figure 20-10.** **(A)** Flail P1 scallop of the mitral valve seen in this "superior" home view.

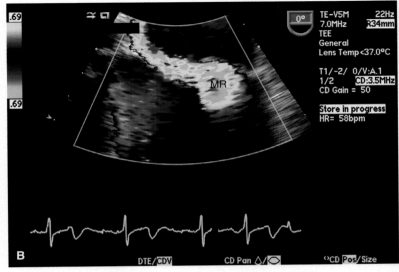

**Figure 20-10.** (*Continued*) **(B)** Severe eccentric anteriorly directed MR.

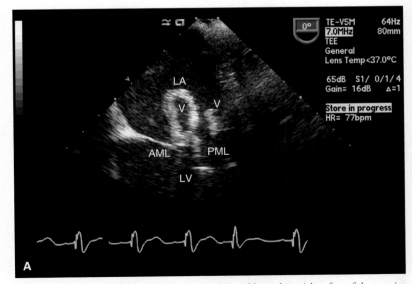

**Figure 20-11. A:** Home view with vegetations (V) visible on the atrial surface of the anterior (AML) and posterior (PML) MV leaflets. (*continued*)

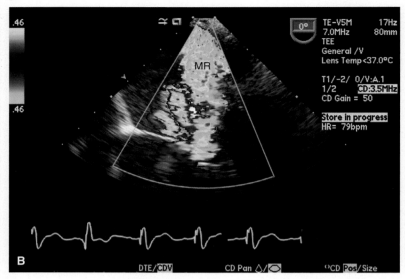

Figure 20-11. (*Continued*) **B:** Severe MR is seen secondary to leaflet malcoaptation and destruction.

## Aortic Valve

See Figures 20-12–20-14.

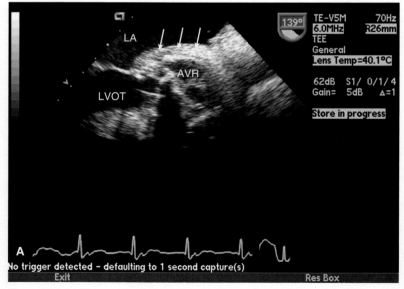

Figure 20-12. (**A**) 120-degree long-axis view showing an aortic mechanical valve with abnormally thickened aortic root suggestive of abscess.

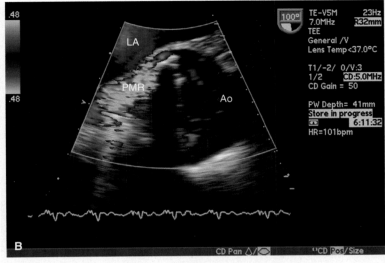

Figure 20-12. (*Continued*) (**B**) Perivalvular regurgitation.

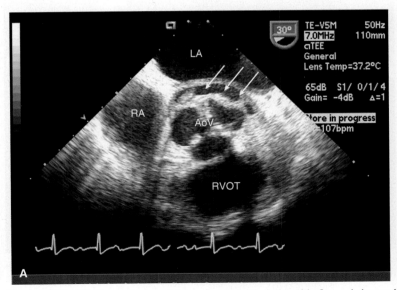

Figure 20-13. (**A**) Short-axis view of the aortic valve with thickened leaflets and abnormal fluid (*arrows*) seen in the supporting aortic root tissue. (*continued*)

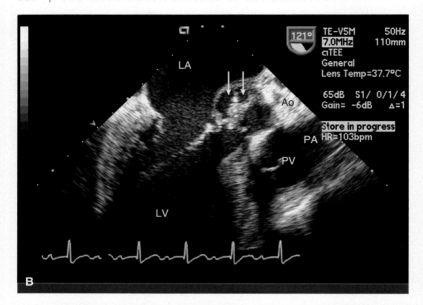

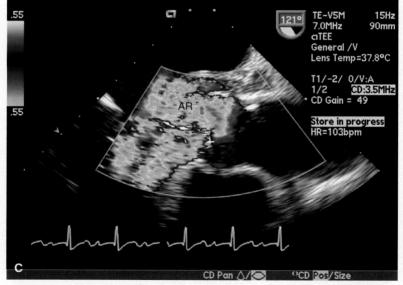

**Figure 20-13.** (*Continued*) (**B**) Long-axis LV view confirms aortic root abscess (*arrows*) with (**C**) severe AR.

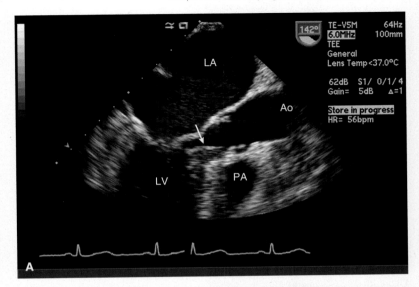

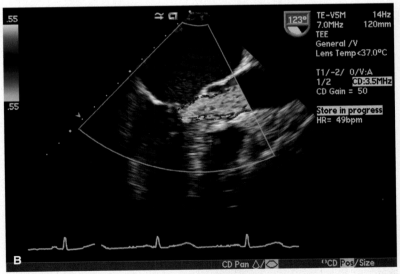

Figure 20-14. (A) Long-axis LV view with narrowing of the LVOT secondary to tunnel type subaortic membrane (*arrow*). (B) Marked systolic turbulence is seen in the LVOT (C) and mild AR. (*continued*)

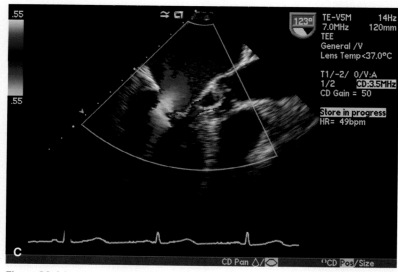

Figure 20-14. (*Continued*)

## Aorta

See Figures 20-15–20-17.

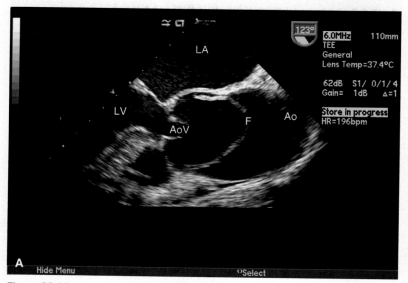

Figure 20-15. Dissection flap seen in the aortic root on a (A) long-axis and (B) short-axis view.

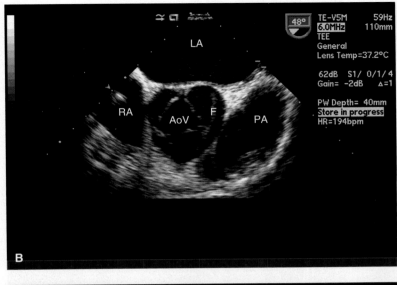

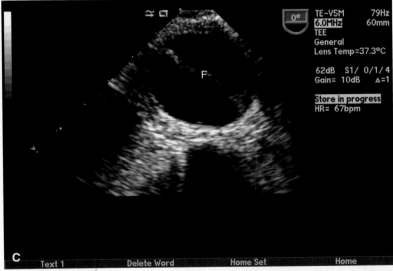

Figure 20-15. (*Continued*) The dissection flap extended to the descending thoracic aorta (**C**).

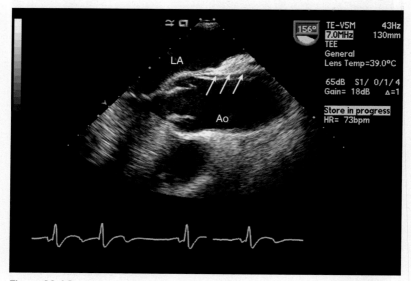

**Figure 20-16.** View of the aortic root showing abnormal fluid in the wall of the proximal ascending aorta consistent with intramural hematoma (*arrows*).

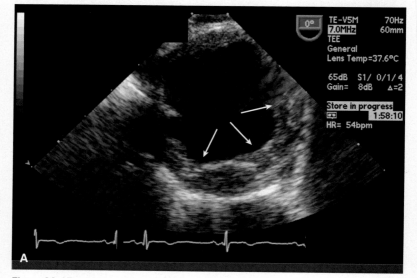

**Figure 20-17.** (**A**) Short-axis and (**B**) long-axis view of significant aortic atheroma seen in the descending thoracic aorta (*arrows*).

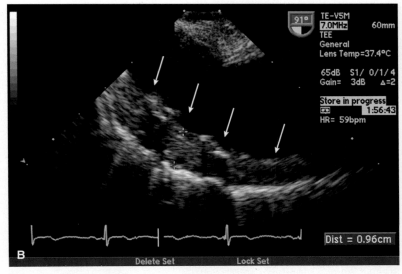

**Figure 20-17.** (*Continued*)

## Thrombus in Transit
See Figure 20-18.

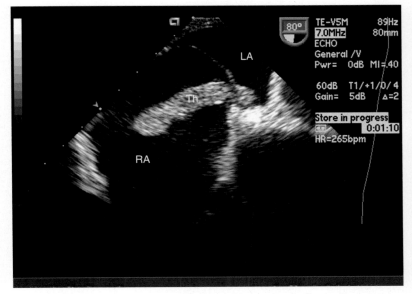

**Figure 20-18.** Thrombus seen crossing the interatrial septum at the fossa ovalis.

## LAA Thrombus

See Figure 20-19.

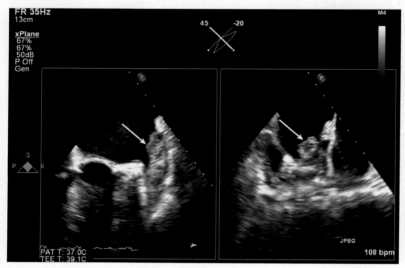

**Figure 20-19.** Biplanar view of LAA thrombus (*arrows*). Spontaneous echo contrast can be seen in the LA.

# Index

Note: Page numbers followed by f and t indicates figure and table respectively.